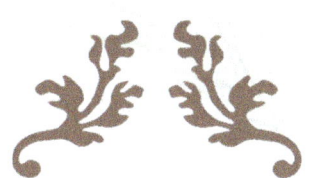

ALZHEIMER'S DIET COOKBOOK FOR SENIORS 2024

Delicious Recipes to Support Brain Health and Well-Being

DR. JEFFREY M. WALTER

DR. JEFFREY M. WALTER

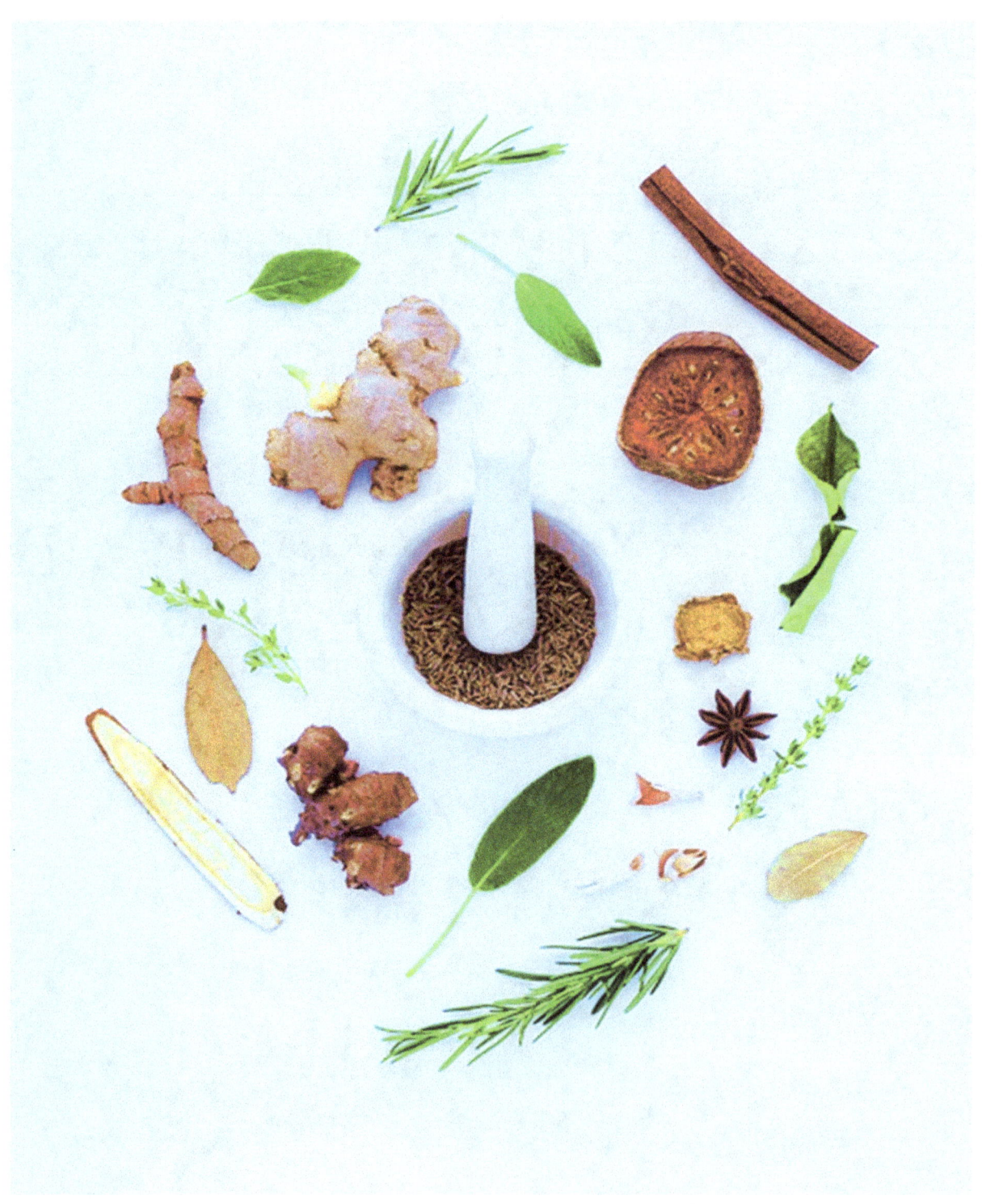

DR. JEFFREY M. WALTER

All right reserved. No part of this publication should be reproduced, distributed, or transmitted in any form or by any means, including photocopying, recording, or other electronic or mechanical methods, without the prior written permission of the publisher, except in the case of brief quotations embodied in critical reviews and certain other noncommercial uses permitted by copyright law.

Copyright@ Dr. Jeffrey M. Walter, 2024.

DR. JEFFREY M. WALTER

Contents

Introduction 5
    Comprehending Alzheimer's Disease and Diet 5
    The Significance of Nutrients for Brain Health 5
    Role of balanced diet's 6
    MIND Nutrition 6
    Useful Advice for Adopting a Brain-Healthy Diet 6
    The Caregiver's Role in Alzheimer's Diet 7
    Diet's Impact on Alzheimer's Disease 8
    Essential Elements for Mental Wellness 8
    Hazardous food ingredients 9
    Alzheimer's disease and nutritional habits 9
    MIND Nutrition 10
    Useful Advice for a Brain-healthy Diet 10
    The Support Caregivers Provide for a Diet That Is Brain-Healthy 11
    Advice for Seniors Using the Kitchen 11

Breakfast Recipes 16
    Breakfast Recipes: A Nutritious Start to the Day 17
    Highlights of Our Breakfast Recipes: 17

Lunch Recipes 24
    Lunch Recipes: Nourishing Meals for Sustained Energy 25

Dinner Recipes 33
    Dinner Recipes: Wholesome Evening Meals for Optimal Health 34

Snack Recipes 42
    Snack Recipes: Healthy and Energizing Bites 43

Dessert Recipes 49
    Dessert Recipes: Sweet Treats for a Balanced Diet 50

Beverage Recipes 57
    Beverages: Refreshing and Nourishing Drinks 58

Meal Plan 65

Meal Plan 66

14-Days Meal Plan 68

ADVICE FOR SENIORS AND FAMILIES 70

Wrapping up 72
    Motivation to Maintain a Healthy Diet 72

DR. JEFFREY M. WALTER

Introduction
Comprehending Alzheimer's Disease and Diet

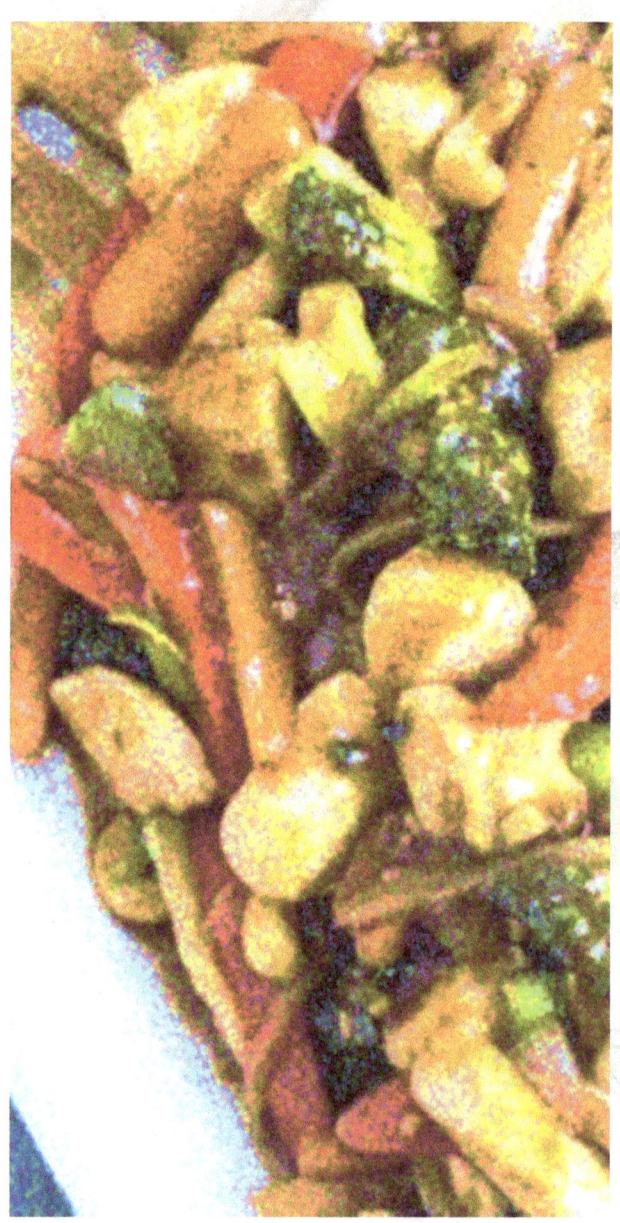

The Link Between Diet and Alzheimer's Disease

Alzheimer's disease is a neurological illness that worsens over time and is marked by behavioral abnormalities, memory loss, and cognitive deterioration. It continues to be among the most prevalent types of dementia, impacting millions of elderly people globally. Although there isn't a recognized treatment for Alzheimer's, several lifestyle choices, such as nutrition and food, are very important in controlling the disease's symptoms and perhaps delaying its course.

The Significance of Nutrients for Brain Health

In addition to being vital for preserving general health and well-being, nutrition is especially important for brain function. Nutrients that promote cognitive function and may lower the risk of Alzheimer's disease are advantageous. Among these nutrients are:

1. Omega-3 fatty acids

Omega-3 fatty acids are very essential nutrients for all Alzheimer patients. They may be found in flaxseeds, walnuts, chia seeds, and seafood like salmon, mackerel, and sardines. They lessen oxidative stress, promote cognitive health, and preserve the composition and functionality of brain cells.

2. Antioxidants

Free radical damage is prevented by antioxidants such as beta-carotene, vitamins C and E, and beta-carotene. Antioxidant-rich foods, including berries, leafy green vegetables, nuts, and seeds, may support the preservation of cognitive function.

3. Vitamin-B complex

The B vitamins are essential for healthy brain function, including folate (B9), B6, and B12. They help lower homocysteine levels, which are associated with a deterioration in cognitive function. Legumes, eggs, fortified cereals, and leafy greens are excellent sources of B vitamins.

4. Vitamin D

Both general health and brain function depend on vitamin D. A higher risk of cognitive deterioration has been linked to low vitamin D levels. Vitamin D may be obtained via sunshine, fatty fish, and fortified dairy products.

5. Polyphenols

It has been shown that polyphenols, which are present in foods like berries, dark chocolate, tea, and red wine, have neuroprotective properties. By lowering inflammation and encouraging normal blood flow to the brain, they enhance brain function.

Role of balanced diet's

Cognitive health may be considerably improved by eating a balanced diet that includes certain nutrients that are good for the brain. The benefits of several dietary regimens for Alzheimer's disease have been investigated; the MIND (Mediterranean-DASH Diet Intervention for Neurodegenerative Delay) and Mediterranean diets have shown the most promise.

Dietary Mediterranean

The Mediterranean diet places a strong emphasis on eating plenty of fruits, vegetables, whole grains, legumes, nuts, seeds, and olive oil. It also calls for consuming dairy products, fish, and chicken in moderation, as well as limiting sweets and red meat. This diet is beneficial for the health of the brain since it is high in polyphenols, antioxidants, and omega-3 fatty acids.

MIND Nutrition

The DASH (Dietary Approaches to Stop Hypertension) and Mediterranean diets are combined in the MIND diet. Ten food categories are highlighted as being beneficial to the brain: whole grains, fish, poultry, olive oil, berries, nuts, green leafy vegetables, and wine (in moderation). Limiting foods that are bad for the brain, such as red meat, butter and margarine, cheese, pastries, and fried or fast food, is another key component of the MIND diet.

Useful Advice for Adopting a Brain-Healthy Diet

Putting into practice a brain-healthy diet entails developing mindful eating practices and attentive dietary choices. The following useful advice is intended for elders and caregivers:

1. Prioritize fresh foods.

Opt for whole, fresh foods rather than packaged and processed ones. The cornerstones of your diet should consist of entire grains, lean meats, fresh produce, and healthy fats.

2. Arrange a balanced diet.

Try to eat meals that are well-balanced and rich in different nutrients. Include whole grains, lean protein, and veggies at every meal to guarantee that you are getting a balanced supply of vital nutrients.

3. Maintain hydration.

Cognitive function may be adversely affected by dehydration. Along with eating a diet rich in hydrating foods like fruits and vegetables, make sure you receive enough water throughout the day.

4. Cut back on saturated fats and sugar.

Consuming too much sugar and saturated fat may lead to oxidative stress and inflammation, both of which are detrimental to the health of the brain. Reduce your intake of sugary snacks, sweets, and meals high in saturated fats.

5. Add nutrition-boosting snacks.

Select brain-boosting foods such as yogurt, berries, almonds, and seeds. These nutrient-rich snacks promote general health and cognitive function.

The Caregiver's Role in Alzheimer's Diet

To maintain the general health and nutrition of people with Alzheimer's disease, caregivers are essential. Seniors' quality of life may be positively impacted by ensuring that meals are wholesome, tasty, and catered to their requirements.

1. Planning and preparing meals

To maintain a balanced diet and lower stress levels, schedule meals in advance. Maintaining consistency in eating habits may also be facilitated by meal preparation in advance.

2. Establishing a Cozy Dining Setting

Establish a serene and cozy dining space. To make eating pleasurable, reduce distractions, deliver meals at regular intervals, and provide help when required.

3. Adapting to meet new needs

As Alzheimer's disease worsens, people may notice changes in their taste, appetite, and ability to swallow. Be flexible and patient; serve meals more often and in smaller portions, modifying the texture of the food as necessary.

To manage the symptoms and promote general brain health, it is essential to comprehend the relationship between diet and Alzheimer's disease. Seniors and their caregivers may significantly improve cognitive performance and quality of life by consuming brain-healthy foods, maintaining a balanced diet, and adopting practical eating habits. It's becoming more evident how crucial nutrition is to preserving brain function as we learn more about the connection between food and Alzheimer's disease.

Diet's Impact on Alzheimer's Disease

Alzheimer's Disease

Millions of individuals worldwide are impacted by the progressive neurological illness known as Alzheimer's disease. It is the most prevalent form of dementia in older people, characterized by behavioral abnormalities, disorientation, and memory loss. As the illness worsens, there is a significant loss of cognitive function and an inability to carry out everyday tasks. Although the precise etiology of Alzheimer's disease remains uncertain, a confluence of genetic, environmental, and behavioral factors is thought to be responsible. Nutrition, in particular, has become one of the most important areas of research for Alzheimer's disease treatment and prevention.

The Impact of Food on Brain Health

Like the rest of the body, the brain needs healthy nourishment to perform at its best. Our brain's structure and function may be influenced by the foods we eat, which can affect everything from cognitive function to the likelihood of acquiring neurodegenerative disorders like Alzheimer's. While certain nutrients may hurt cognitive function, others are very advantageous for brain health.

Essential Elements for Mental Wellness

The Fatty Acids Omega-3:

- Sources: walnuts, chia seeds, flaxseeds, and fatty fish (sardines, mackerel, and salmon).
- Benefits: DHA (docosahexaenoic acid), in particular, is an omega-3 fatty acid that is essential for preserving the integrity and functionality of neuronal membranes. They are linked to a lower incidence of cognitive deterioration and have anti-inflammatory qualities.

Oxidants

- Sources: dark chocolate, green leafy vegetables, berries, nuts, and seeds.
- Benefits: Free radicals, the source of oxidative stress in the brain, are countered by antioxidants. The aging process and the emergence of neurodegenerative disorders are both significantly influenced by oxidative stress.

Vitamin B:

- Sources: nuts, leafy greens, legumes, dairy products, eggs, and whole grains.
- Benefits: The health of the brain depends on B vitamins, especially B6, B12, and folate. They assist in lowering blood homocysteine levels, which are linked to a higher risk of Alzheimer's disease when they are raised.

Vitamin D

- Sources: supplements, fatty fish, sunshine, and fortified dairy products.
- Benefits: The formation and operation. Vitamin D deficiency has been associated with a higher incidence of Alzheimer's disease and cognitive impairment.

Polyphenols:

- Sources: tea, red wine, dark chocolate, fruits (particularly berries), and vegetables.
- Benefits: Polyphenols can protect neurons. They boost cognitive function by lowering inflammation and enhancing blood flow to the brain.

Hazardous food ingredients

Trans and Saturated fats:

- Sources: margarine, baked products, fried foods, and processed foods.
- Impact: Diets high in trans and saturated fats cause increased oxidative stress and inflammation, which may exacerbate cognitive impairment.

Refined Sugars and Carbohydrates:

- Sources: white bread, soda, sugary snacks, and desserts.
- Risk factors for Alzheimer's disease include obesity, elevated oxidative stress, insulin resistance, and a high intake of refined sugars and carbs.

Drinking too much alcohol:

- Impact: Drinking too much alcohol over an extended period may harm the brain and raise the risk of dementia. Because red wine contains a lot of polyphenols, moderate consumption of it may provide some protection.

Alzheimer's disease and nutritional habits

Studies have shown that certain eating habits may impact an individual's likelihood of getting Alzheimer's disease. Two of the diets that have been researched and suggested for brain health are the Mediterranean diet and the MIND (Mediterranean-DASH Diet Intervention for Neurodegenerative Delay) diet.

Dietary Mediterranean

- Eating whole, minimally processed foods is emphasized in the Mediterranean diet. Examples of these items are:
- Fruits and vegetables are rich in vitamins, minerals, and antioxidants.
- Whole grains offer vital nutrients and long-lasting energy.
- Legumes are rich in protein and fiber.
- Nuts and seeds are excellent sources of protein, antioxidants, and good fats.
- One of the main sources of beneficial monounsaturated fats is olive oil.
- Rich sources of omega-3 fatty acids include fish and seafood.
- Cheese and yogurt, in particular, are moderate dairy products.
- Less Red Meat: Emphasizes chicken and other lean proteins.
- Red wine is usually drunk with meals and in moderation.

According to studies, following a Mediterranean diet lowers the risk of Alzheimer's disease and cognitive decline. The diet's focus on foods high in antioxidants and anti-inflammatory properties promotes general health, including brain function.

MIND Nutrition

Combining elements of the DASH (Dietary Approaches to Stop Hypertension) and Mediterranean diets, the MIND diet emphasizes brain-healthy foods while minimizing those that are harmful to cognitive function. The MIND diet includes the following:

- Consume at least six servings of green leafy vegetables each week.
- One dish or more of other vegetables per day.
- Five servings of nuts each week.
- Beans: a minimum of three servings per week.
- Eat three or more servings
- Fish: one dish per week at the very least.
- Poultry: two meals or more per week, at the very least.
- Olive is the main cooking oil.
- One glass of wine every day, if desired.

Limiting items like red meat, cheese, butter, and margarine, pastries and sweets, and fried or fast food is another key component of the MIND diet. Studies show that even a modest follower of the MIND diet may considerably lower their chance of developing Alzheimer's disease.

Useful Advice for a Brain-healthy Diet

Making wise decisions and forming enduring eating habits are key components of putting a brain-healthy diet into practice. Here are a few useful pointers:

1. Give fresh foods a priority.

Eat more fresh meals as opposed to packaged and processed stuff.

2. Arrange well-balanced meals.

Make sure a variety of nutrients are included in each meal. To make balanced, nutrient-dense meals, include veggies, lean protein, whole grains, and healthy fats.

3. Maintain hydration.

Cognitive function may be impacted by dehydration. Along with eating a diet rich in hydrating foods like fruits and vegetables, make sure you receive enough water throughout the day.

4. Limit sugar and unhealthy fats.

Limit your consumption of processed carbohydrates, trans fats, and saturated fats. These may raise the risk of cognitive impairment by causing oxidative stress and inflammation.

5. Add nutrition-boosting snacks.

Choose brain-boosting foods like yogurt, berries, almonds, and seeds. These nutrient-dense foods promote cognitive performance.

6. Prepare food at home.

When you cook at home, you have more control over the ingredients and portion quantities. It also offers a chance to try out different brain-healthy cooking ideas.

DR. JEFFREY M. WALTER

The Support Caregivers Provide for a Diet That Is Brain-Healthy

Caregivers are essential in helping people with Alzheimer's disease have a diet that is beneficial for their brains. Among their duties are:

1. Planning and preparing meals

To guarantee a well-rounded and nourishing diet, schedule and prepare meals in advance. Meal preparation in advance may also help preserve consistency and lower stress levels.

2. Establishing a Satisfying Dining Ambience

Establish a serene and cozy dining space. To make eating pleasurable, reduce distractions, deliver meals at regular intervals, and provide help when required.

3. Adapting to meet new needs

As Alzheimer's disease worsens, people may notice changes in their taste, appetite, and ability to swallow. In addition to providing smaller, more frequent meals and modifying the texture of food as necessary, caregivers must be flexible and patients.

It is critical to conduct research and provide practical applications in nutrition and Alzheimer's disease. People and those who provide care for them may make educated food decisions that promote cognitive function and general well-being by knowing how nutrition affects brain health. The MIND and Mediterranean diets provide helpful guidelines for including foods that are good for the brain in everyday meals, which may lower the risk of Alzheimer's disease and halt its development. Individuals with Alzheimer's disease may be able to improve their quality of life with careful food choices and healthy nourishments.

Advice for Seniors Using the Kitchen

Organizing and getting ready

Organizing Meals:
- Make a food plan in advance to guarantee a healthy, well-balanced diet.
- Incorporate whole grains, lean meats, fruits, veggies, and healthy fats into your diet plan.
- Purchasing groceries:
- To prevent making pointless purchases, create a shopping list based on your scheduled meals.
- Select fresh foods over processed ones.

Prepare Ahead:
- Prepare ingredients in advance by washing and cutting vegetables.
- Make bigger amounts of food and store some in the freezer for later use.

Make recipes simpler:

Select recipes that don't take a lot of steps or are simple to make.

To save time, use frozen or pre-cut veggies.

Cooking Techniques

- Use Nutritious Cooking Techniques:
- Instead of frying, try baking, steaming, grilling, or sautéing.
- Use non-stick cookware to reduce the need for extra fats.
- Add ingredients high in nutrients:
- Increase the amount of veggies in casseroles, stews, and soups.
- Make use of entire grains, such as whole wheat pasta, brown rice, and quinoa.
- Taste But Not Too Much Salt:
- Spices, herbs, garlic, and lemon juice may all be used to boost taste without using salt.
- Try using salt-free substitutes and spice combinations.

Make food appealing.

- Be mindful of how food is presented; use eye-catching plating and vibrant veggies.
- To establish a schedule, serve meals at the same time every day.

Assisting Seniors

Promote Involvement:

- As much as possible, get the elders involved in meal planning and preparation.
- Assign basic chores like measuring, stirring, and arranging the table.
- Be kind and patient.
- Recognize that eating and cooking might take longer and that you might need extra help.
- Encourage others and show patience when difficulties come up.

Adjust for Tastes and Capabilities:

- Observe the nutritional requirements and food preferences of the elderly.
- If chewing or swallowing are problems, adjust the food's texture.
- Establish a relaxing dining space.
- Make sure there are no distractions and that the eating space is peaceful.
- Make use of cozy chairs and suitable table arrangements.

Seniors' Safety in the Kitchen

Generally Safe Advice

- Uncluttered and well-organized space:
- Make sure all the paths are clear and the kitchen is clutter-free.
- To save needless bending and straining, keep commonly used things close at hand.
- Sufficient Lighting
- To lower the chance of mishaps, make sure the kitchen is well-lit.
- For surfaces like stovetops and counters where precise work is done, use task lighting.

Non-Slip Surfaces:

- To stop falls, use rugs or non-slip mats.
- To prevent slips, make sure the floors are spotless and dry.

User-Friendly Appliances:

- Select appliances with straightforward controls and large, readable buttons.
- Make sure every appliance functions properly and, if at all feasible, has an automated shut-off option.
- When cooking, be safe.

Monitoring and Support:

- Seniors should never be left alone in the kitchen, particularly while using the stove or oven.
- Help with the handling of hot utensils, pots, and pans.

Safe Management of Hot Objects:

- When handling hot cookware, put on oven gloves or potholders.
- Use heat-resistant mats or trivets to place hot goods on solid surfaces.

How to Prevent Burns and Scalds:

- To avoid unintentional tipping, turn the pot handles inside out on the burner.
- Before serving, check the temperature of the food and beverages to prevent burns.

Fire Safety:

- Learn how to use a fire extinguisher and keep one handy in the kitchen.
- When cooking, stay away from wearing loose clothes since they might catch fire.

Safety When Using Knives

Using knives properly:

- Make use of knives with well-grip ergonomic handles.
- Knives should always be kept sharp to minimize the power required to cut.

Safe Cutting Methods:

- To keep your cutting board from sliding, choose one that is sturdy and cover it with a moist towel.
- When cutting, keep your fingers curled under and cut away from the body.

Storage of knives:

- To avoid mishaps, keep knives in a dedicated knife block or drawer with blade guards.
- Knives should not be left in the sink where they cannot be seen.
- Electrical Security

Utilizing Electrical Appliances Safely:

- Check for damage to electrical cables and repair them as needed.
- When plugging appliances directly in, replace extension cables with wall outlets.

Preventing Overloads

- Don't put too many gadgets in one electrical outlet at once.
- When not in use, unplug small equipment to reduce the danger of electrical fires.

Dietary safety

Correct storage of food:

- Make sure the refrigerator is set at the proper temperature and store perishables inside as soon as possible.
- To make sure leftovers are eaten or thrown out on time, label and date them.

Handling food safely:

- Both before and after handling food, properly wash your hands.

- To avoid cross-contamination, keep raw meats and other items on different cutting boards.

Heating food to safe levels:

- To make sure meats are cooked to safe internal temperatures, use a food thermometer.
- To eliminate any possible germs, reheat leftovers to the proper temperatures.

It takes care and initiative in the kitchen to guarantee the security and dietary health of elderly people, especially those suffering from Alzheimer's disease. Through knowledge of essential nutrients for brain health, caregivers may choose foods that promote cognitive performance. Caregivers may provide wholesome and enticing meals for their patients by putting these helpful meal planning, preparation, and cooking methods into practice. Setting kitchen safety as a top priority also helps avoid mishaps and guarantees a safe space for elders to eat. Caregivers who work together can greatly improve seniors' quality of life by fostering their physical and emotional well-being.

DR. JEFFREY M. WALTER

RECIPES

1 Breakfast Recipes

DR. JEFFREY M. WALTER

Breakfast Recipes: A Nutritious Start to the Day

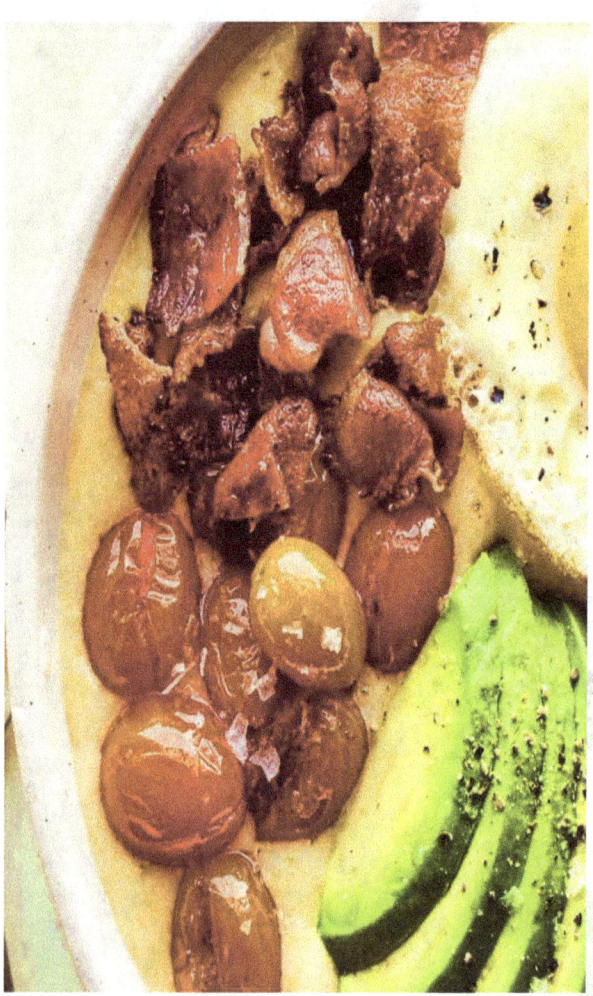

Breakfast is often considered the most important meal of the day, especially for seniors managing Alzheimer's disease. A nutritious breakfast can provide essential nutrients to kickstart brain function, improve concentration, and boost overall energy levels. Our selection of breakfast recipes in this cookbook focuses on incorporating brain-healthy ingredients that are both delicious and easy to prepare. These recipes are designed to meet the dietary needs of seniors, ensuring a balanced intake of proteins, healthy fats, whole grains, and fresh fruits and vegetables.

Highlights of Our Breakfast Recipes:

- **Blueberry Oatmeal with Walnuts:** A hearty and fiber-rich oatmeal topped with antioxidant-packed blueberries and brain-boosting walnuts.
- **Spinach and Mushroom Frittata:** A protein-rich frittata loaded with spinach and mushrooms, providing essential vitamins and minerals.
- **Avocado and Berry Smoothie:** A creamy and refreshing smoothie that combines the healthy fats of avocado with the antioxidants of mixed berries.
- **Greek Yogurt with Honey and Almonds:** A simple yet satisfying breakfast featuring protein-packed Greek yogurt, sweetened with a touch of honey and crunchy almonds.
- **Chia Seed Pudding with Fresh Berries:** An overnight pudding made with nutrient-dense chia seeds, topped with a variety of fresh berries for a burst of flavor and color.

Each recipe is crafted to be both nutritious and appealing, helping seniors start their day on a healthy and positive note.

1. Blueberry Oatmeal with Walnuts

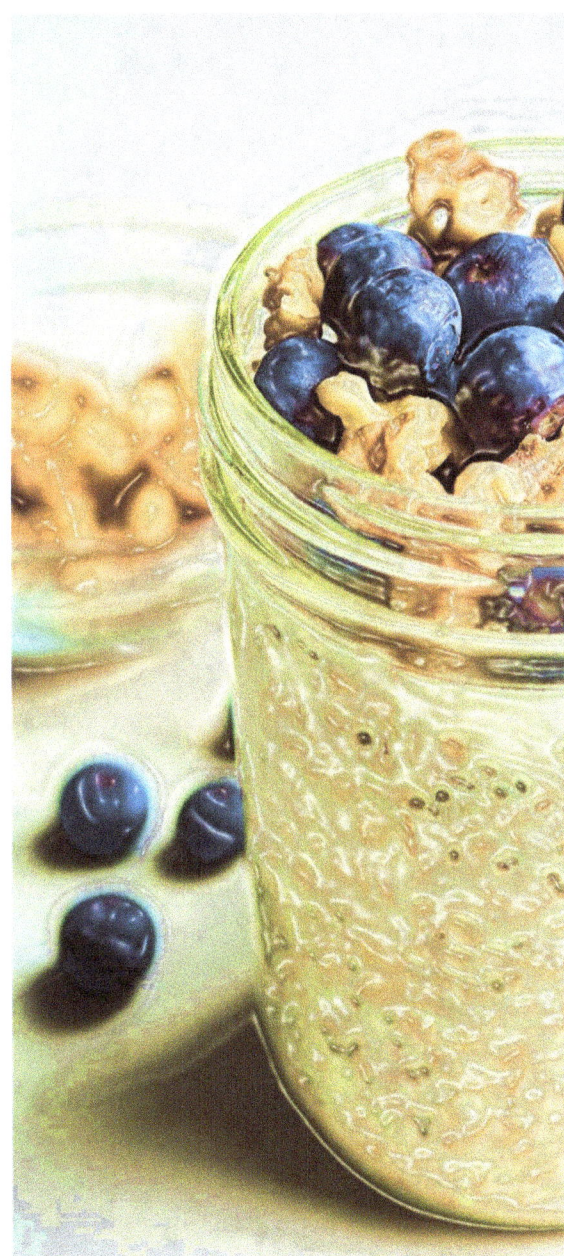

- Time of Preparation: 5 minutes
- Cooking Time: 10 minutes
- Servings: 2

Ingredients

- 1 cup rolled oats
- Two cups of water or you can use milk.
- 1 cup fresh or frozen blueberries
- 1/4 cup chopped walnuts
- 1 tablespoon honey or maple syrup (optional)
- 1/2 teaspoon ground cinnamon
- Pinch of salt

Procedure

- Heat the milk or water in a medium saucepan until it begins to boil.
- After adding the rolled oats, lower the heat to a medium level.
- Cook, stirring periodically, until the oats are tender and the liquid is absorbed, approximately 5 minutes.
- Stir in the cinnamon, walnuts, blueberries, and a little amount of salt. Mix well to blend.
- Cook the blueberries for a further two to three minutes, or until they are thoroughly cooked.
- After turning off the heat, let the oatmeal take a minute to settle.
- If preferred, serve warm with a honey or maple syrup drizzle.

Nutritional Values (per serving)

- Calories: 320
- Protein: 8g
- Carbohydrates: 50g
- Fiber: 8g
- Sugars: 12g
- Fat: 12g
- Omega-3 fatty acids: 2.5g

Cooking Tips

- Add a splash of milk or a dollop of yogurt on top for extra creaminess.

- Substitute walnuts with almonds or pecans if preferred.

Health Benefits

- Antioxidants: Blueberries are rich in antioxidants, which help protect brain cells from oxidative damage.
- Healthy Fats: Walnuts provide omega-3 fatty acids that support brain health.
- Fiber: Oats are high in fiber, promoting digestive health and stable blood sugar levels.

2. Spinach and Mushroom Frittata

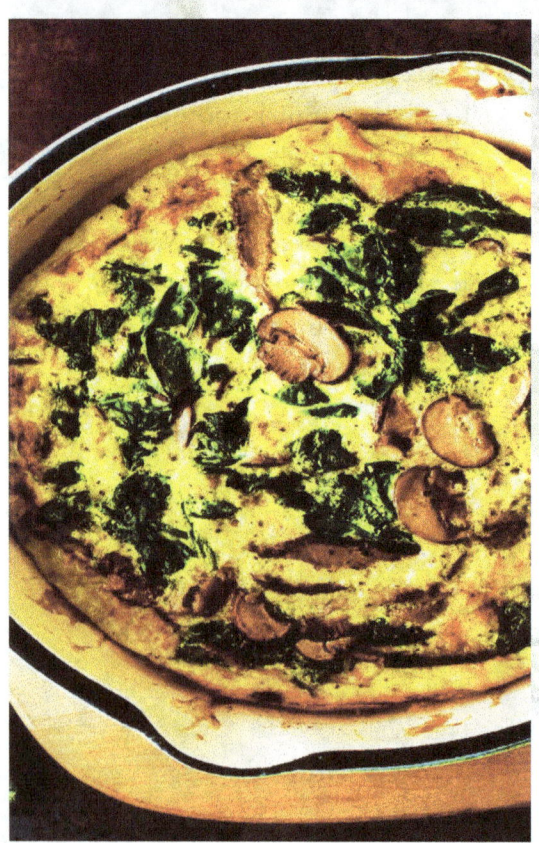

- Time of Preparation: 10 minutes
- Cooking Time: 20 minutes
- Servings: 4

Ingredients

- 6 large eggs
- 1/4 cup milk (dairy or non-dairy)
- 1 cup fresh spinach, chopped
- 1 cup mushrooms, sliced
- 1/2 cup shredded cheese (optional)
- 1 small onion, finely chopped
- 1 clove garlic, minced
- 2 tablespoons olive oil
- Salt and pepper to taste

Procedure

- Set the oven's temperature to 175°C/350°F.
- Stir and mix milk and eggs together. Add pepper and salt for seasoning.
- In a skillet that is oven safe, preheat the olive oil over medium heat.
- Add the onion and garlic, and cook for approximately 3 minutes, or until transparent.
- Add the mushrooms and simmer for approximately 5 minutes, or until they shed their moisture and begin to brown.
- Add the spinach and simmer, stirring, for approximately 2 minutes, or until wilted.
- Over the veggies in the pan, pour the egg mixture. If using, sprinkle with cheese.
- Cook until the edges begin to firm, 3 to 4 minutes on the burner.

- After placing the pan in the oven, bake it for ten to twelve minutes, or until the frittata is well cooked and has a golden brown top.
- Take it out of the oven and give it a little time to cool down before slicing and serving.

Nutritional Values (per serving)

- Calories: 180
- Protein: 12g
- Carbohydrates: 5g
- Fiber: 1.5g
- Sugars: 2g
- Fat: 12g

Cooking Tips

- Use a non-stick or well-seasoned cast-iron skillet to prevent sticking.
- Substitute spinach with kale or Swiss chard if preferred.
- Add a variety of vegetables like bell peppers or zucchini for more flavor and nutrients.

Health Benefits

- Protein: Eggs provide high-quality protein essential for muscle repair and overall health.
- Vitamins and Minerals: Spinach and mushrooms are rich in vitamins and minerals, supporting overall wellness.
- Low Carb: This frittata is low in carbohydrates, making it a great option for maintaining stable blood sugar levels.

3. Avocado and Berry Smoothie

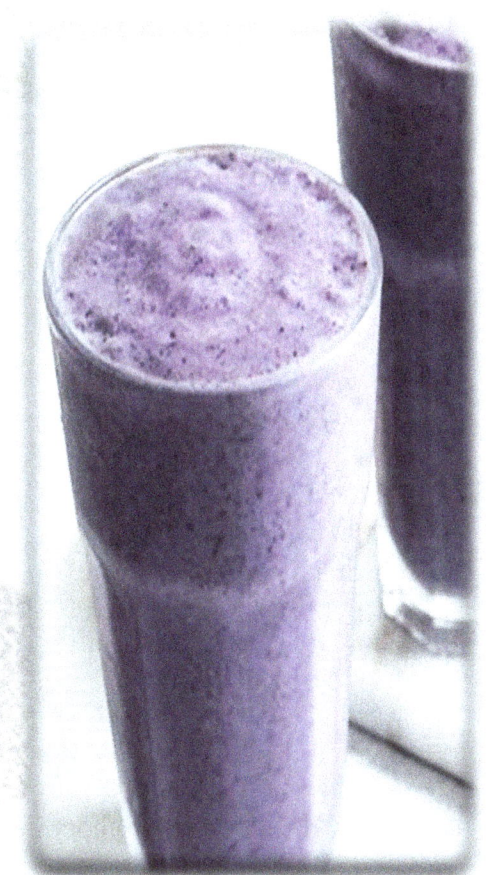

- Time of Preparation: 5 minutes
- Cooking Time: 0 minutes
- Servings: 2

Ingredients

- 1 ripe avocado
- 1 cup mixed berries (blueberries, strawberries, raspberries)
- 1 cup spinach or kale (optional)
- 1 banana
- One cup of almond milk
- 1 tablespoon chia seeds
- 1 teaspoon honey or maple syrup (optional)

Procedure

- Halve the avocado, remove the pit, then scoop out the flesh to put in a blender.
- Add the chia seeds, banana, almond milk, mixed berries, and spinach or kale, if using.
- Process on high until creamy and smooth.
- If you want it sweeter, taste and add more honey or maple syrup.
- Transfer into glasses and serve right away.

Nutritional Values (per serving)

- Calories: 250
- Protein: 4g
- Carbohydrates: 35g
- Fiber: 10g
- Sugars: 15g
- Fat: 12g

Cooking Tips

- To make a thicker, cooler smoothie, use frozen fruit.
- Add more or less milk to adjust the consistency.
- For added protein, include a scoop of protein powder or a spoonful of Greek yogurt.

Health Benefits

- Healthy Fats: Avocado provides monounsaturated fats that are good for heart and brain health.
- Antioxidants: Berries are high in antioxidants, which help fight oxidative stress.
- Fiber: Chia seeds and spinach add extra fiber, supporting digestive health.

4. Greek Yogurt with Honey and Almonds

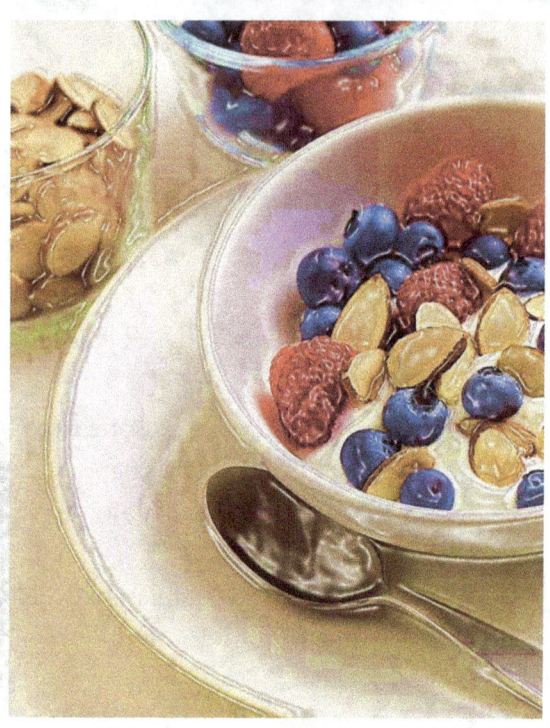

- Time of Preparation: 5 minutes
- Cooking Time: 0 minutes
- Servings: 2

Ingredients

- 1 cup Greek yogurt (plain or vanilla)
- 2 tablespoons honey
- 1/4 cup sliced almonds
- 1/2 teaspoon ground cinnamon
- Fresh fruit (optional, for topping)

Procedure

- Divide the Greek yogurt into two serving bowls.
- Pour one spoonful of honey into each bowl.
- Sprinkle the sliced almonds and ground cinnamon on top.
- Add fresh fruit like berries, banana slices, or apple chunks if desired.
- Serve immediately.

Nutritional Values (per serving)

- Calories: 220
- Protein: 15g
- Carbohydrates: 20g
- Fiber: 2g
- Sugars: 18g
- Fat: 10g

Cooking Tips

- Toast the almonds in a dry skillet for a few minutes to enhance their flavor.
- Experiment with different nuts and seeds for variety.

Health Benefits

- Protein: Greek yogurt is an excellent source of protein, aiding in muscle maintenance and repair.
- Probiotics: Yogurt contains probiotics that support gut health.
- Healthy Fats: Almonds provide healthy fats and additional protein.

5. Chia Seed Pudding with Fresh Berries

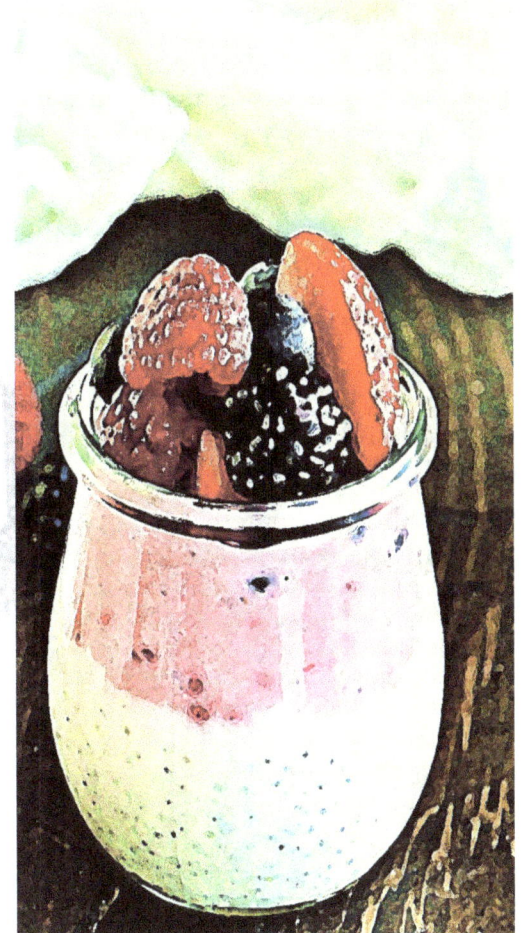

- Time of Preparation: 5 minutes
- Cooking Time: 0 minutes (overnight soaking)
- Servings: 2

Ingredients

- 1/4 cup chia seeds
- One cup almond milk

- 1 tablespoon honey or maple syrup
- 1/2 teaspoon vanilla extract
- 1 cup fresh berries (strawberries, blueberries, raspberries)

Procedure

- Mix the chia seeds, almond milk, honey, and vanilla essence in a medium-sized bowl.
- The mixture should thicken to a pudding-like consistency after at least 4 hours or overnight in the refrigerator, covered.
- Stir the pudding before serving and divide it into two bowls.
- Top each serving with fresh berries.
- Proceed to serve

Nutritional Values (per serving)

- Calories: 200
- Protein: 5g
- Carbohydrates: 30g
- Fiber: 12g
- Sugars: 15g
- Fat: 8g

Cooking Tips

- Stir the pudding a few times during the first hour of soaking to prevent clumping.
- Use any type of milk (dairy or non-dairy) according to your preference.

Health Benefits

- Fiber: Chia seeds are a great source of fiber, aiding in digestion.
- Omega-3 Fatty Acids: Chia seeds provide plant-based omega-3s that support brain health.

2 Lunch Recipes

DR. JEFFREY M. WALTER

Lunch Recipes: Nourishing Meals for Sustained Energy

These recipes incorporate a variety of wholesome ingredients to promote brain health and provide a balanced meal for seniors. From hearty salads to comforting soups, each recipe is designed to deliver both flavor and nourishment, ensuring seniors feel energized and satisfied throughout the day.

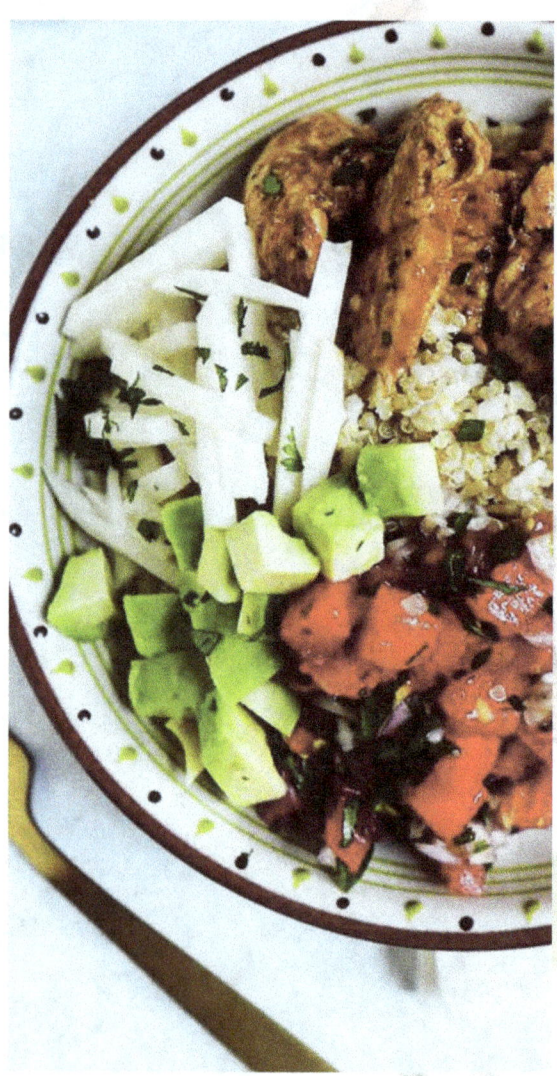

Lunch is a vital part of the day, providing essential nutrients to maintain energy levels and support overall well-being, especially for seniors managing Alzheimer's disease. Our collection of lunch recipes in this cookbook focuses on delicious and nutrient-rich dishes that are easy to prepare and satisfying to enjoy.

1. Quinoa Salad with Kale and Cranberries

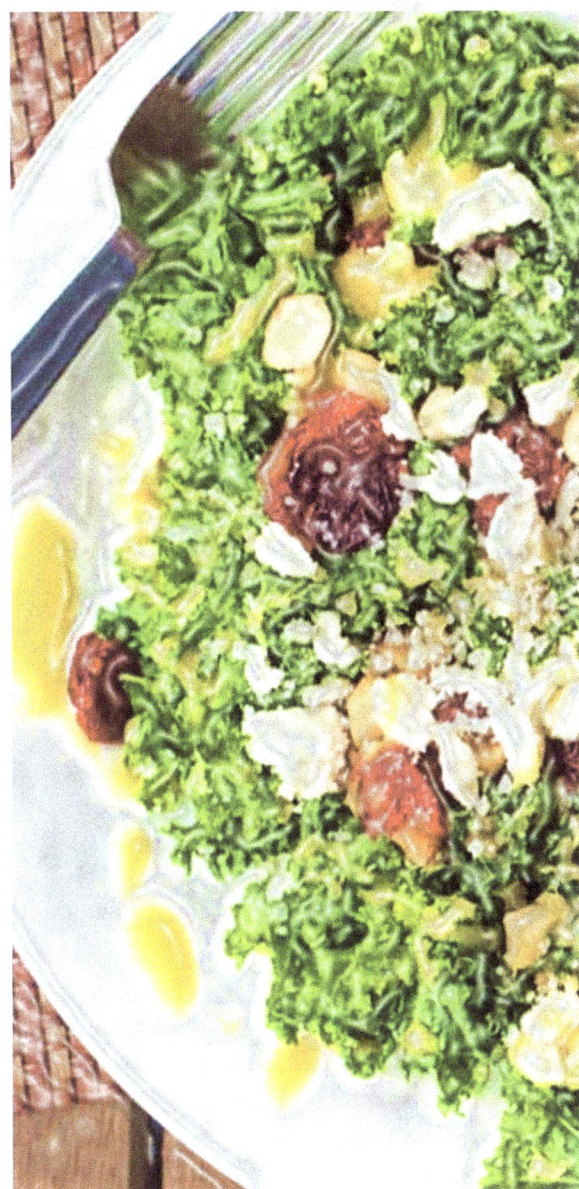

- Time of Preparation: 15 minutes
- Cooking Time: 20 minutes
- Servings: 4

Ingredients

- 1 cup quinoa
- 2 cups water or vegetable broth
- 2 cups chopped kale
- 1/2 cup dried cranberries
- 1/4 cup chopped walnuts
- 1/4 cup crumbled feta cheese (optional)
- 2 tablespoons olive oil
- 1 tablespoon apple cider vinegar
- 1 tablespoon lemon juice
- Salt and pepper to taste

Procedure

- Wash the quinoa in cool water.
- Boil the vegetable broth in a saucepan. After adding the quinoa, lower the heat, cover, and simmer until the water is absorbed—about 15 minutes.
- After turning off the heat, leave the quinoa covered for five minutes. Using a fork, fluff.
- The cooked quinoa, chopped kale, walnuts, dried cranberries, and feta cheese, if used, should all be combined in a big bowl.
- Mix the olive oil, lemon juice, apple cider vinegar, salt, and pepper in a small bowl.
- After adding the dressing to the quinoa mixture, toss to blend.
- In order to let the flavors mingle, serve right away or chill for an hour.

Nutritional Values (per serving)

- Calories: 290
- Protein: 8g
- Carbohydrates: 38g
- Fiber: 5g
- Sugars: 10g
- Fat: 12g

Cooking Tips

- Massage the kale with a little olive oil before adding it to the salad to make it more tender.
- Use any variety of quinoa you prefer: white, red, or black.

Health Benefits

Fiber: Quinoa and kale are excellent sources of dietary fiber, aiding digestion and maintaining blood sugar levels.

- Antioxidants: Dried cranberries and kale are rich in antioxidants, which protect brain cells from oxidative damage.
- Healthy Fats: Walnuts provide essential omega-3 fatty acids that support brain health.

2. Lentil Soup with Carrots and Celery

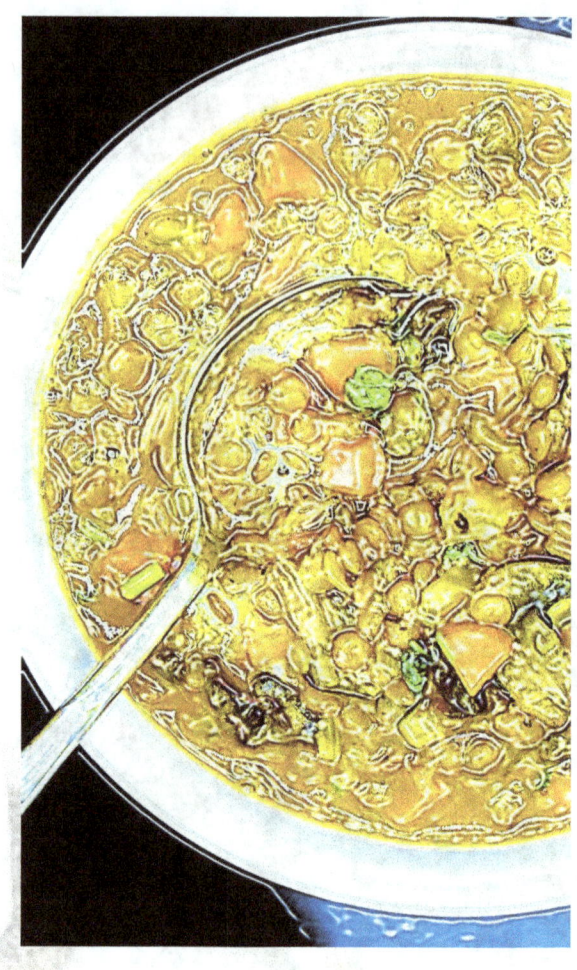

- Time of Preparation: 15 minutes
- Cooking Time: 40 minutes
- Servings: 6

Ingredients

- 1 cup dry, rinsed lentils, either brown or green
- 1 large onion, chopped
- 3 carrots, peeled and chopped
- 3 celery stalks, chopped
- 3 cloves garlic, minced
- 6 cups vegetable broth
- 1 can (14.5 oz) diced tomatoes
- 1 teaspoon dried thyme
- 1 teaspoon ground cumin

- 1 bay leaf
- 2 tablespoons olive oil
- Salt and pepper to taste
- Fresh parsley, chopped (optional, for garnish)

Procedure

- Warm the olive oil
- Add the onion, carrots, and celery, and cook until the vegetables are softened, about 10 minutes.
- Stir in the garlic, thyme, and cumin, and cook for another 1-2 minutes until fragrant.
- Add the lentils, vegetable broth, diced tomatoes, and bay leaf. Bring to a boil.
- Once the lentils are soft, reduce the heat to low, cover, and simmer for 30 to 35 minutes.
- Season with salt and pepper to taste.
- Remove bay leaf before serving.
- Garnish with chopped parsley if desired.

Nutritional Values (per serving)

- Calories: 180
- Protein: 10g
- Carbohydrates: 30g
- Fiber: 10g
- Sugars: 6g
- Fat: 3g

Cooking Tips

- Substitute green or brown lentils with red lentils for a quicker cooking time and different texture.

Health Benefits

- Protein: Lentils are an excellent plant-based protein source, supporting muscle health and repair.
- Fiber: Lentils, carrots, and celery provide high fiber content, promoting digestive health and stable blood sugar levels.
- Vitamins and Minerals: This soup is rich in vitamins A, C, and K, along with iron and folate, essential for overall health.

3. Grilled Chicken and Avocado Wrap

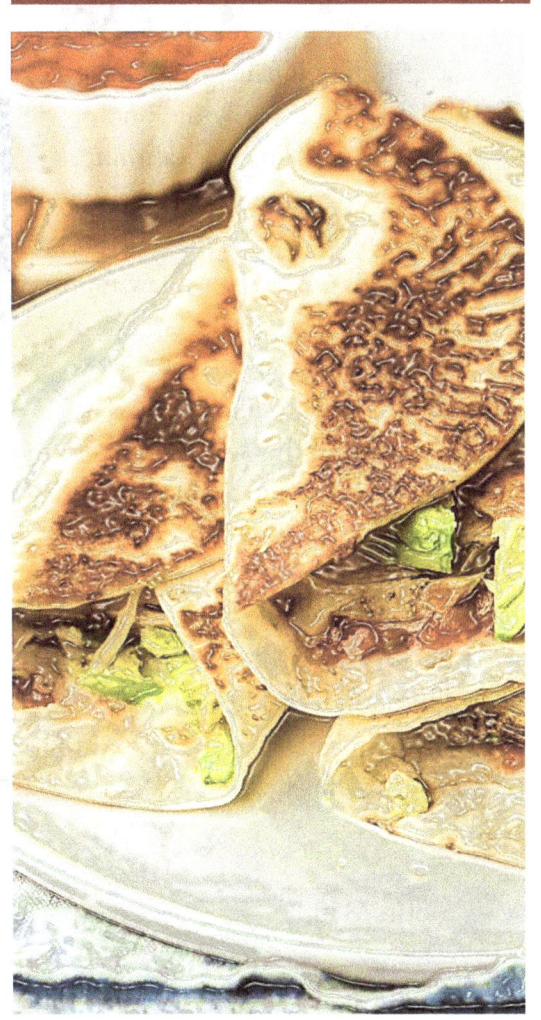

- Time of Preparation: 10 minutes
- Cooking Time: 15 minutes
- Servings: 4

Ingredients

- 2 boneless, skinless chicken breasts
- 2 avocados, sliced
- 1 cup cherry tomatoes, halved
- 1/4 cup red onion, thinly sliced
- 4 whole wheat tortillas
- 1/4 cup plain Greek yogurt
- 2 tablespoons lime juice
- 1 tablespoon olive oil
- Salt and pepper to taste

Procedure

- Turn the heat up to medium-high on the grill or grill pan.
- Add a little olive oil, salt, and pepper to the chicken breasts' seasoning.
- Grill for 6-7 minutes on each side, or until the chicken is cooked through. After letting it rest for a few minutes, cut it thinly.
- In a small bowl, mix the Greek yogurt and lime juice to make a dressing.
- To assemble the wraps, lay out the tortillas and spread a tablespoon of the yogurt dressing on each.
- Add slices of avocado, grilled chicken, cherry tomatoes, and red onion.
- Roll up the tortillas tightly, securing with toothpicks if needed.
- Serve immediately, or wrap in foil for a portable lunch.

Nutritional Values (per serving)

- Calories: 350
- Protein: 25g
- Carbohydrates: 30g
- Fiber: 8g
- Sugars: 3g
- Fat: 15g

Cooking Tips

- Marinate the chicken in a mixture of lime juice, garlic, and cumin for extra flavor before grilling.
- Use a grill pan or skillet if an outdoor grill is not available.
- Substitute Greek yogurt with hummus or avocado spread if preferred.

Health Benefits

- Protein: Grilled chicken provides lean protein, essential for muscle maintenance and repair.
- Healthy Fats: Avocado offers monounsaturated fats that are beneficial for heart and brain health.
- Fiber: Whole wheat tortillas and vegetables add fiber, supporting digestion and satiety.

4. Roasted Beet and Goat Cheese Salad

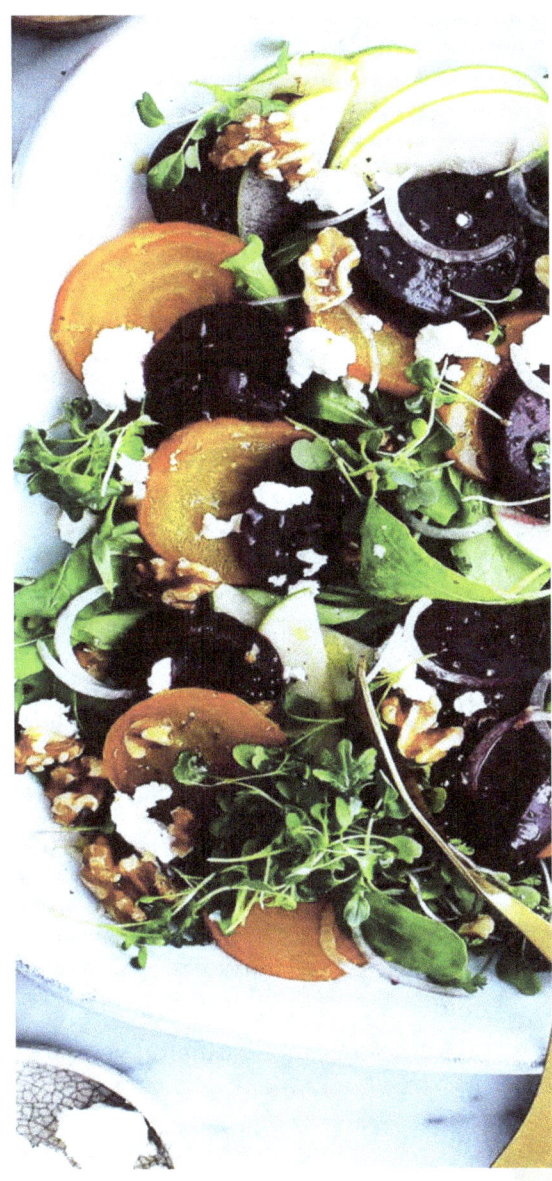

- Time of Preparation: 15 minutes
- Cooking Time: 45 minutes
- Servings: 4

Ingredients

- 4 medium beets, peeled and diced
- 2 tablespoons olive oil
- 4 cups mixed greens (arugula, spinach, or mixed salad greens)
- 1/4 cup crumbled goat cheese
- 1/4 cup walnuts, toasted
- 2 tablespoons balsamic vinegar
- Salt and pepper to taste

Procedure

- Preheat the oven to 400°F (200°C).
- Add salt, pepper, and olive oil to the diced beets. Spread on a baking sheet.
- Roast in the oven for 35-45 minutes, turning once, until beets are tender and slightly caramelized.
- Let the beets cool slightly before assembling the salad.
- In a large bowl, combine the mixed greens, roasted beets, goat cheese, and walnuts.
- Drizzle with balsamic vinegar and toss gently to combine.
- Serve immediately.

Nutritional Values (per serving)

- Calories: 220
- Protein: 6g
- Carbohydrates: 22g
- Fiber: 5g
- Sugars: 14g
- Fat: 14g

Cooking Tips

- Use pre-cooked beets to save time on roasting.
- Add slices of apple or pear for extra sweetness and texture.
- Substitute goat cheese with feta or blue cheese if preferred.

Health Benefits

- Antioxidants: Beets are high in antioxidants, which help protect against oxidative stress.

- Healthy Fats: Walnuts provide omega-3 fatty acids, supporting brain health.

Vitamins and Minerals: Mixed greens and beets are rich in vitamins A, C, and K, along with folate and iron.

5. Tomato Basil Soup with Whole Grain Bread

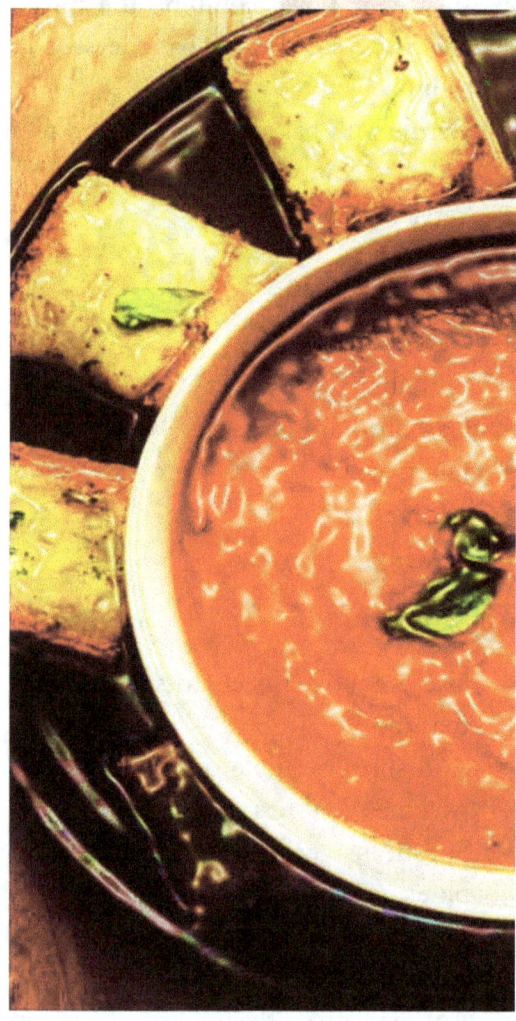

- Time of Preparation: 10 minutes
- Cooking Time: 30 minutes
- Servings: 4

Ingredients

- 2 tablespoons olive oil
- 1 medium onion, chopped
- 3 cloves garlic, minced
- 2 cans (28 oz each) crushed tomatoes
- 2 cups vegetable broth
- 1/4 cup fresh basil leaves, chopped
- 1 teaspoon dried oregano
- Salt and pepper to taste
- Whole grain bread, for serving

Procedure

- Heat the olive oil in a suitable sauce pan
- Add the chopped onion and simmer for approximately 5 minutes, or until softened.
- Once fragrant, stir in the garlic and simmer for an additional one to two minutes.
- Add the oregano, basil, and vegetable broth along with the smashed tomatoes. Heat till boiling.
- After lowering the heat to low, simmer for 20 minutes.
- Puree the soup using an immersion blender until it's smooth, or gently transfer it to a blender and process in stages.
- To taste, add salt and pepper for seasoning.
- Warm up and accompany with pieces of whole grain bread.

Nutritional Values (per serving)

- Calories: 180

- Protein: 5g
- Carbohydrates: 25g
- Fiber: 6g
- Sugars: 12g
- Fat: 7g

Cooking Tips

- Add a splash of cream or milk for a creamier soup.
- Use fresh tomatoes during peak season for a more robust flavor.
- Garnish with additional fresh basil or a drizzle of olive oil before serving.

Health Benefits

- Antioxidants: Tomatoes are rich in lycopene, an antioxidant that helps protect against cell damage.
- Fiber: Whole grain bread provides dietary fiber, aiding digestion and maintaining blood sugar levels.
- Vitamins and Minerals: This soup is an excellent source of vitamins A and C, supporting immune function and skin health.

3 Dinner Recipes

DR. JEFFREY M. WALTER

Dinner Recipes: Wholesome Evening Meals for Optimal Health

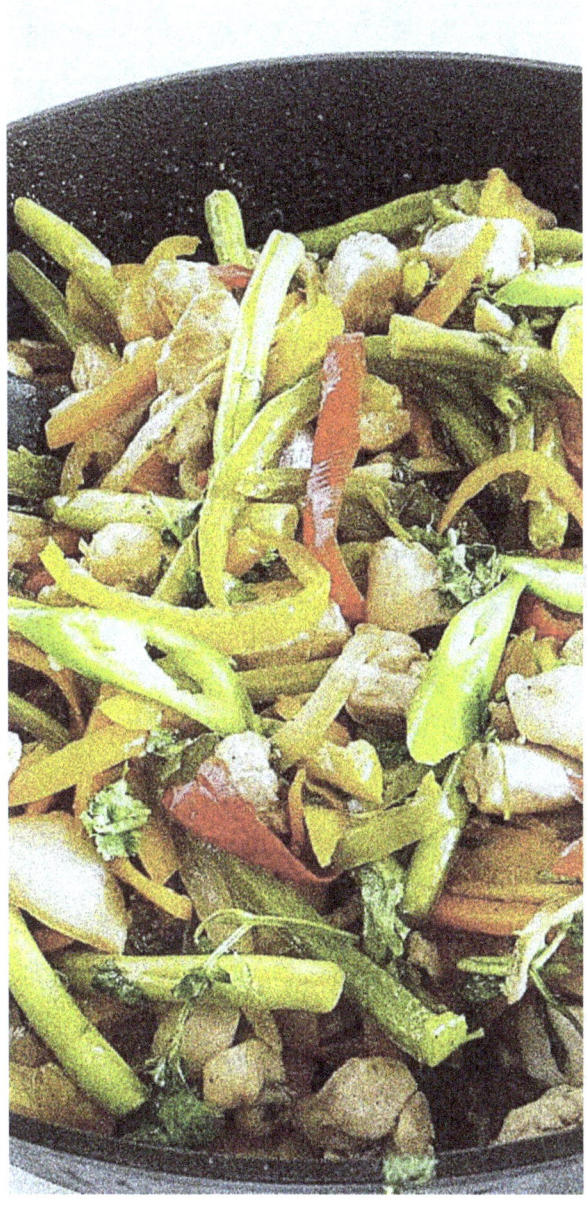

Dinner is a crucial meal that helps seniors maintain their energy levels and supports overall health as they wind down for the day. Our dinner recipes are designed to be both nutritious and satisfying, ensuring a balanced intake of proteins, healthy fats, and vital nutrients. These recipes are created with simplicity in mind, making them easy to prepare while still delivering robust flavors and nourishing ingredients. From hearty main dishes to comforting sides, our dinner recipes aim to promote brain health, improve cognitive function, and provide a delightful end to the day.

DR. JEFFREY M. WALTER

1. Baked Salmon with Asparagus

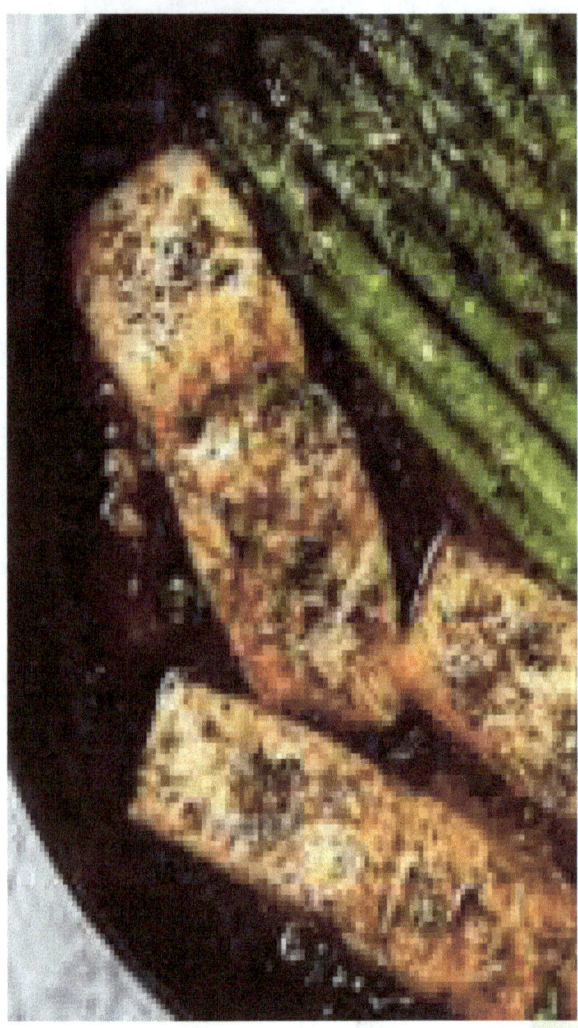

- Time of Preparation: 10 minutes
- Cooking Time: 20 minutes
- Servings: 4

Ingredients

- 4 salmon fillets (about 6 oz each)
- 1 bunch asparagus, trimmed
- 2 tablespoons olive oil
- 1 lemon, sliced
- 2 cloves garlic, minced
- 1 teaspoon dried dill
- Salt and pepper to taste

Procedure

Preheat the oven to 400°F (200°C).

Place the salmon fillets on a parchment paper-lined baking pan.

Arrange the asparagus, cut side down, around the fish.

Pour some olive oil over the asparagus and fish.

Season the salmon and asparagus with salt, pepper, dried dill, and chopped garlic.

Put a slice of lemon on a filet

Bake in the preheated oven for 20 minutes, or until the salmon flakes easily with a fork and the asparagus is tender.

Serve immediately.

Nutritional Values (per serving)

- Calories: 350
- Protein: 35g
- Carbohydrates: 5g
- Fiber: 2g
- Sugars: 2g
- Fat: 20g

Cooking Tips

- For an extra burst of citrus, squeeze additional lemon juice over the dish before serving.

Health Benefits

- Omega-3 Fatty Acids: Salmon is rich in omega-3s, essential for brain health and reducing inflammation.

- Vitamins: Asparagus is high in vitamins A, C, and K, supporting immune and bone health.
- Protein: Provides high-quality protein necessary for muscle repair and maintenance.

2. Chicken and Vegetable Stir-Fry

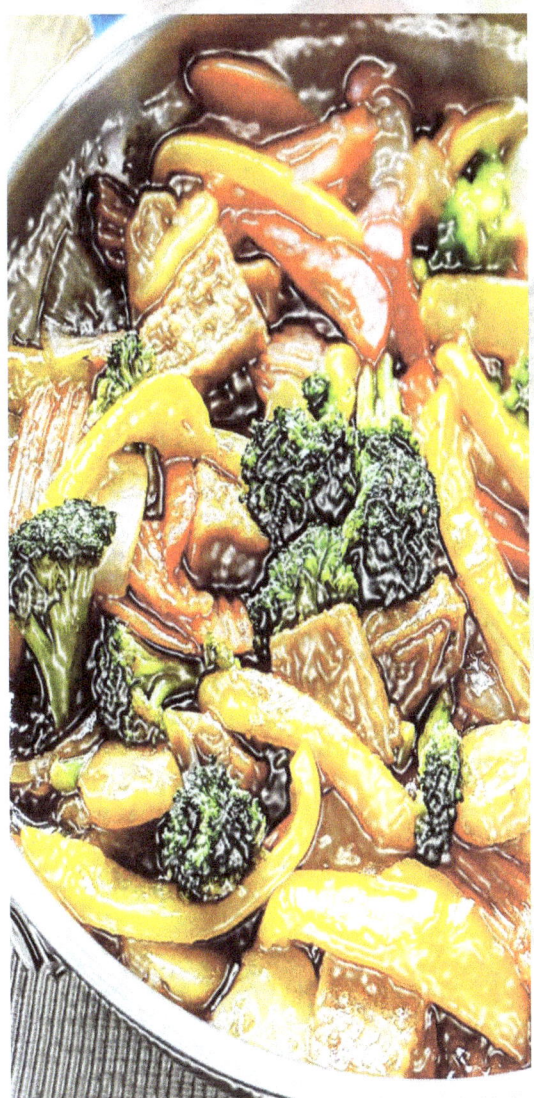

- Time of Preparation: 15 minutes
- Cooking Time: 15 minutes
- Servings: 4

Ingredients

- 1 lb boneless chicken breast
- 2 cups broccoli florets
- 1 red bell pepper, sliced
- 1 yellow bell pepper, sliced
- 1 cup snap peas
- 2 carrots, sliced
- 3 tablespoons of tamari
- 2 tablespoons olive oil
- 1 tablespoon honey
- 2 cloves garlic, minced
- 1 teaspoon grated fresh ginger
- Cooked brown rice or quinoa, for serving

Procedure

- In a large pan or wok, heat 1 tablespoon of olive oil over medium-high heat.
- After adding the sliced chicken breast, sauté it for 5 to 7 minutes, or until it is browned and cooked through. Take out and place aside from the skillet.
- Add olive oil
- Add the ginger and garlic, and sauté until fragrant, approximately 1 minute.
- Add the carrots, snap peas, bell peppers, and broccoli. Sauté the veggies for five to seven minutes, or until they are crisp-tender.
- After cooking, add the chicken back to the skillet.
- Mix together the honey and soy sauce. Stir to guarantee even coating after

pouring over the vegetables and chicken.
- Cook until well heated for another 2 to 3 minutes.
- Serve with cooked quinoa or brown rice.

Nutritional Values (per serving)

- Calories: 350
- Protein: 30g
- Carbohydrates: 30g
- Fiber: 6g
- Sugars: 10g
- Fat: 10g

Cooking Tips

- For a meal that looks better, use a range of vibrant veggies.
- For an additional flavorful layer, add a little amount of sesame oil.
- Substitute chicken with tofu for a vegetarian option.

Health Benefits

- Protein: Chicken provides lean protein essential for tissue repair and muscle maintenance.
- Antioxidants: Vegetables like bell peppers and broccoli are high in antioxidants, promoting cellular health.
- Fiber: High fiber content aids in digestion and helps maintain stable blood sugar levels.

3. Stuffed Bell Peppers with Brown Rice

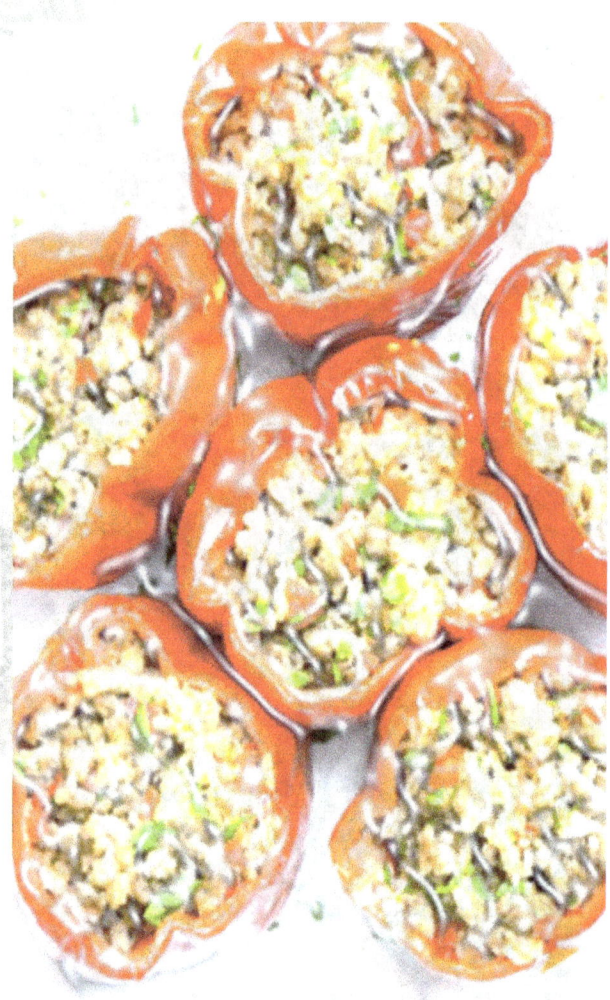

- Time of Preparation: 15 minutes
- Cooking Time: 45 minutes
- Servings: 4

Ingredients

- 4 large bell peppers (any color)
- 1 cup cooked brown rice
- 1 lb ground turkey or beef
- 1 small onion, chopped
- 1 can (15 oz) diced tomatoes, drained
- 1 cup black beans, rinsed and drained
- 1 cup corn kernels (fresh or frozen)
- 1 teaspoon cumin
- 1 teaspoon chili powder
- 1/2 cup shredded cheese (optional)
- Salt and pepper to taste
- Fresh cilantro, chopped (optional, for garnish)

Procedure

- Set the oven to 190°C, or 375°F.
- The bell peppers should be placed vertically in a baking dish.
- Brown the ground beef or turkey in a large pan over medium heat. Remove any extra fat.
- Add the chopped onion and simmer for approximately 5 minutes, or until softened.
- Add the chopped tomatoes, black beans, corn, cumin, chili powder, salt, and pepper, along with the cooked brown rice.
- Filling should be spooned into each bell pepper, packing it very firmly.
- If using, sprinkle some shredded cheese on top.
- Bake the baking dish for thirty minutes with the foil covering it.
- When the peppers are soft and the cheese is melted and bubbling, remove the cover and bake for a further 15 minutes.
- If preferred, garnish with fresh cilantro just before serving.

Nutritional Values (per serving)

- Calories: 400
- Protein: 25g
- Carbohydrates: 50g
- Fiber: 12g
- Sugars: 10g
- Fat: 10g

Cooking Tips

- Use a variety of colored bell peppers for a more vibrant presentation.
- Prepare the filling ahead of time and store it in the refrigerator until ready to stuff the peppers.
- Substitute brown rice with quinoa or cauliflower rice for a different texture and nutritional profile.

Health Benefits

- Fiber: Brown rice, black beans, and bell peppers provide a high fiber content, promoting digestive health.
- Lean Protein: Ground turkey or beef offers lean protein essential for muscle repair and growth.
- Vitamins and Minerals: Bell peppers are rich in vitamins A and C, supporting immune health.

4. Herb-Crusted Cod with Quinoa

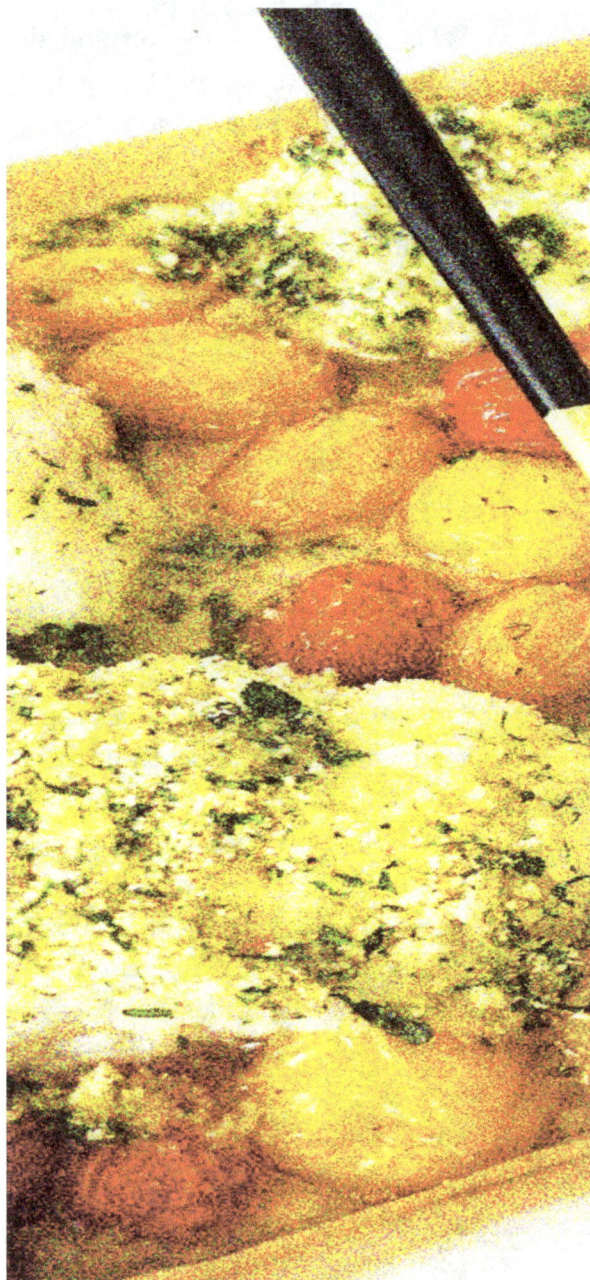

- Time of Preparation: 15 minutes
- Cooking Time: 20 minutes
- Servings: 4

Ingredients

- 4 cod fillets (about 6 oz each)
- 1 cup quinoa
- 2 cups vegetable broth or water
- 1/4 cup fresh parsley, chopped
- 2 tablespoons fresh dill, chopped
- 2 tablespoons fresh chives, chopped
- 2 cloves garlic, minced
- 2 tablespoons olive oil
- 1 lemon, sliced
- Salt and pepper to taste

Procedure

- Set oven temperature to 400°F, or 200°C.
- Wash the quinoa in cool water.
- Heat the water or vegetable broth in a medium-sized pot until it boils. After adding the quinoa, lower the heat, cover, and simmer until the liquid is absorbed—about 15 minutes. Using a fork, fluff and put aside.
- Cod filets should be placed on a baking pan covered with parchment paper.
- Combine the parsley, dill, chives, garlic, olive oil, salt, and pepper in a small bowl.
- Evenly cover the top of each fish filet with the herb mixture.
- Put a slice of lemon on top of each fillet.
- Bake for 15 to 20 minutes, or until a fork can easily pierce the fish, in a preheated oven.

- Over quinoa, serve the herb-crusted fish.

Nutritional Values (per serving)

- Calories: 320
- Protein: 30g
- Carbohydrates: 30g
- Fiber: 5g
- Sugars: 2g
- Fat: 10g

Cooking Tips

- Use fresh herbs for the best flavor; however, dried herbs can be substituted if fresh are not available.
- For added flavor, cook quinoa in vegetable broth instead of water.

Health Benefits

- Omega-3 Fatty Acids: Cod provides omega-3 fatty acids, promoting brain health and reducing inflammation.
- Protein: A high-protein meal supports muscle maintenance and repair.
- Antioxidants: Fresh herbs are packed with antioxidants, supporting overall health.

5. Sweet Potato and Black Bean Enchiladas

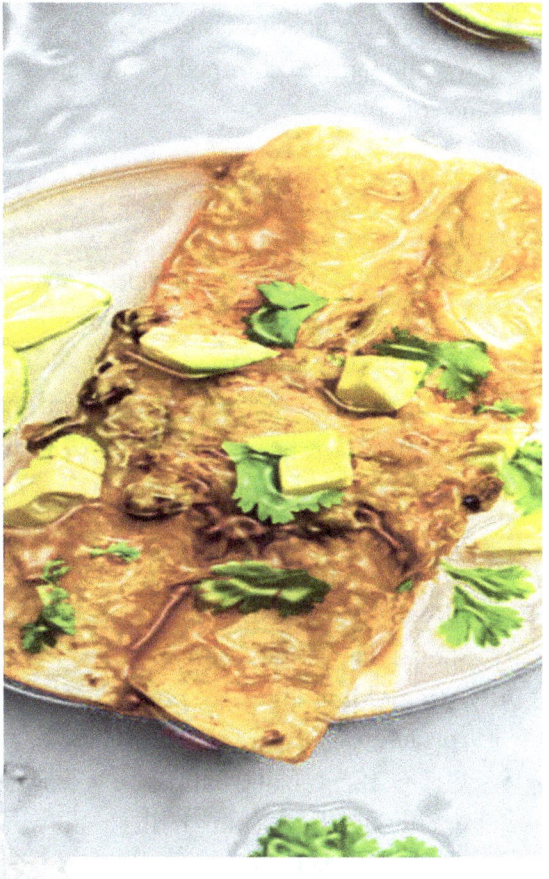

- Time of Preparation: 20 minutes
- Cooking Time: 30 minutes
- Servings: 4

Ingredients

- 2 large sweet potatoes, peeled and diced
- 1 can (15 oz) black beans, rinsed and drained
- 1 cup corn kernels (fresh or frozen)
- 1/2 cup red onion, chopped
- 1/2 cup bell pepper, chopped
- 2 cups enchilada sauce
- 8 small whole wheat tortillas
- 1 cup shredded cheese (optional)
- 2 tablespoons olive oil
- 1 teaspoon cumin
- 1 teaspoon chili powder

- Salt and pepper to taste
- Fresh cilantro, chopped (optional, for garnish)

Procedure

- Heat the olive oil
- After adding the chopped sweet potatoes, simmer for fifteen minutes or until they are soft.
- Add the bell pepper, chili powder, cumin, black beans, corn, red onion, and salt and pepper. Simmer the veggies for a further five minutes, or until they are tender.
- Drizzle a little amount of enchilada sauce in a baking dish.
- After adding the sweet potato mixture to each tortilla, firmly roll each one.
- Cover the tortillas with the leftover enchilada sauce and, if desired, top with shredded cheese.
- Bake the dish for 20 minutes with the foil covering it.
- After removing the foil, bake for a further ten minutes, or until the cheese is bubbling and melted.
- If preferred, garnish with fresh cilantro just before serving.

Nutritional Values (per serving)

- Calories: 380
- Protein: 15g
- Carbohydrates: 60g
- Fiber: 12g
- Sugars: 10g
- Fat: 10g

Cooking Tips

- Use canned enchilada sauce for convenience, or make your own for a fresher flavor.
- For a spicier dish, add a chopped jalapeño to the vegetable mixture.
- Serve with a side of avocado or guacamole for added healthy fats.

Health Benefits

- Fiber: Sweet potatoes and black beans provide high fiber content, promoting digestive health.
- Vitamins and Minerals: Sweet potatoes are rich in vitamins A and C, supporting immune function.
- Protein: Black beans offer plant-based protein essential for muscle repair and growth.

4 Snack Recipes

Snack Recipes: Healthy and Energizing Bites

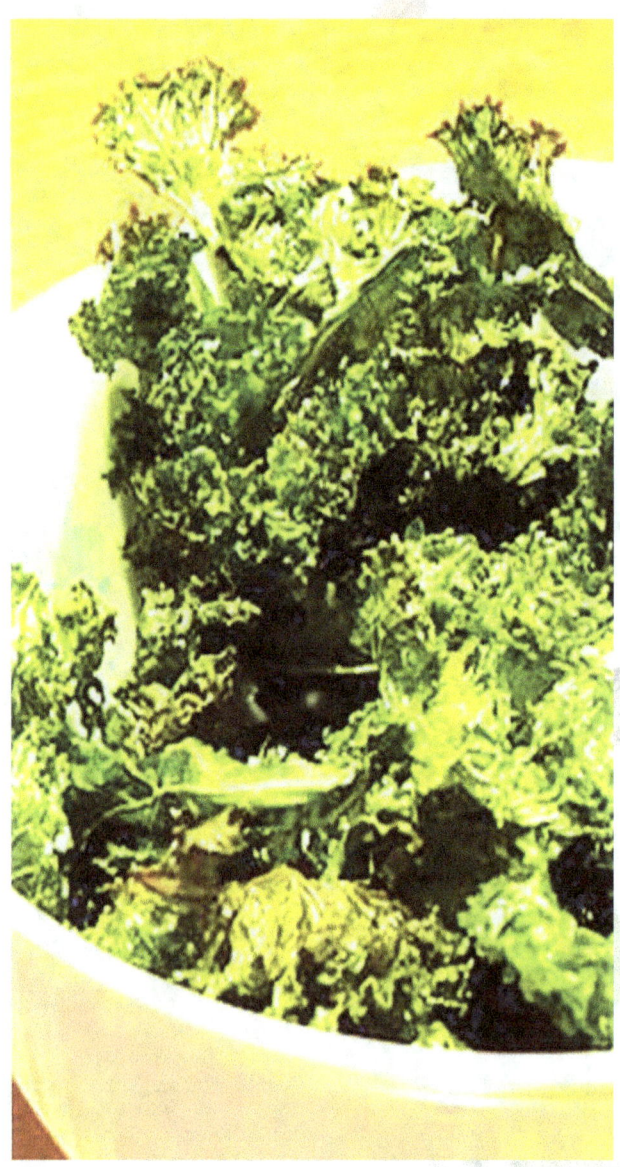

dense options that are easy to prepare and enjoy. These snacks are designed to be both delicious and nutritious, incorporating ingredients known for their brain-boosting properties. From savory bites to sweet treats, our collection of snack recipes ensures that seniors can enjoy a variety of flavors and textures while receiving essential nutrients to support overall health and well-being.

Snacks play a crucial role in maintaining energy levels and supporting cognitive function throughout the day, especially for seniors managing Alzheimer's disease. Our snack recipes focus on providing nutrient-

1. Apple Slices with Almond Butter

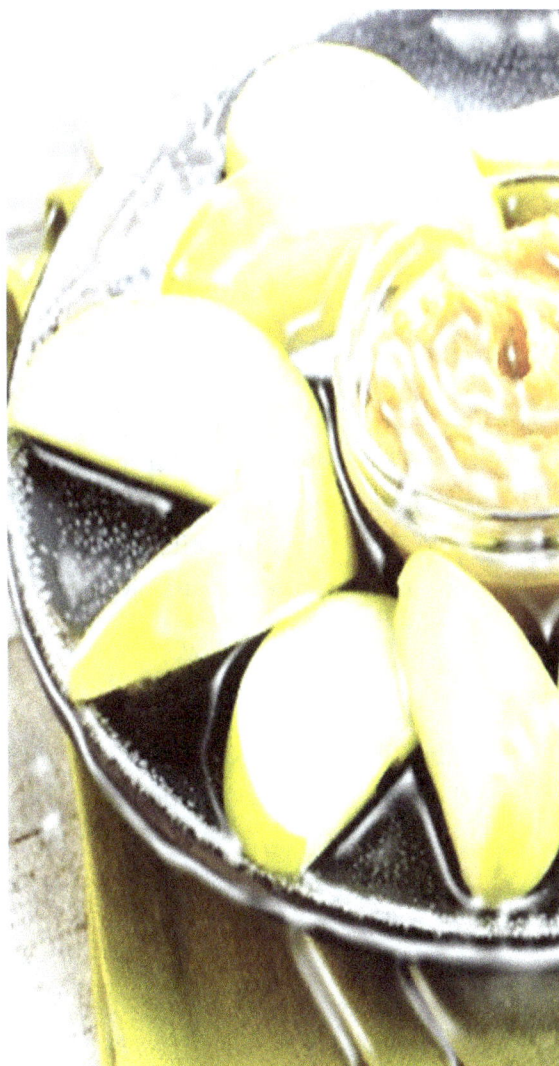

- Time of Preparation: 5 minutes
- Cooking Time: None
- Servings: 2

Ingredients

- 2 medium apples, sliced
- 4 tablespoons almond butter

Procedure

- Wash and core the apples. Cut them into thin slices.
- Arrange the apple slices on a plate.
- Serve with almond butter on the side for dipping.

Nutritional Values (per serving)

- Calories: 230
- Protein: 5g
- Carbohydrates: 28g
- Fiber: 6g
- Sugars: 19g
- Fat: 12g

Cooking Tips

- Choose a variety of apples for different flavors and textures, such as Granny Smith for tartness or Fuji for sweetness.
- Add a sprinkle of cinnamon to the apple slices for extra flavor.

Health Benefits

- Fiber: Apples provide dietary fiber, promoting digestive health and helping to maintain blood sugar levels.
- Healthy Fats: Almond butter offers healthy monounsaturated fats, essential for brain health and reducing inflammation.

2. Hummus with Carrot and Cucumber Sticks

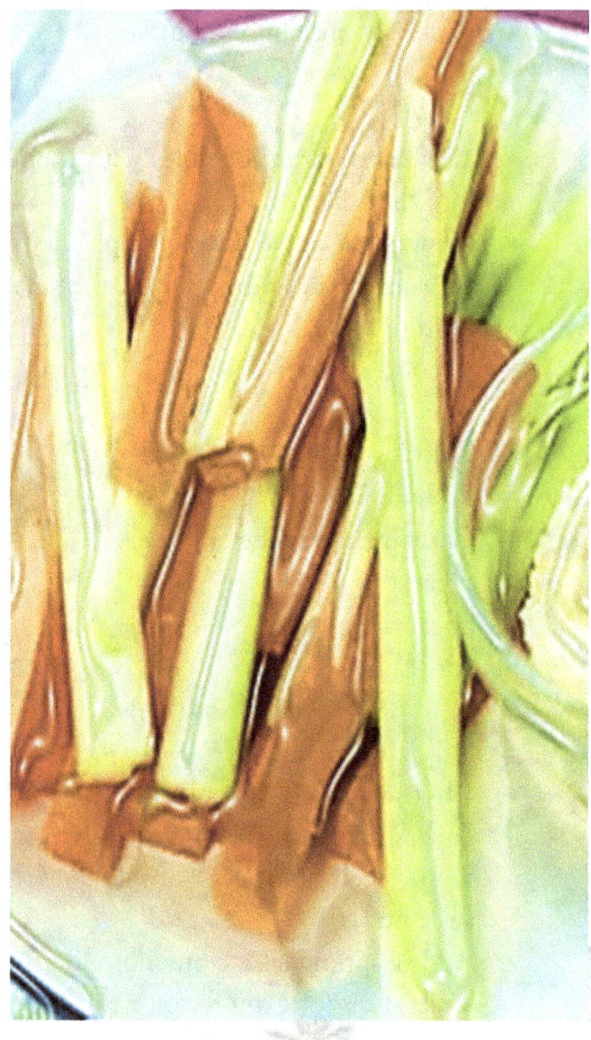

Arrange the vegetable sticks on a plate.

Serve with hummus in a small bowl for dipping.

Nutritional Values (per serving)

- Calories: 100
- Protein: 3g
- Carbohydrates: 12g
- Fiber: 4g
- Sugars: 5g
- Fat: 5g

Cooking Tips

- Make your own hummus for a fresher taste by blending chickpeas, tahini, olive oil, lemon juice, garlic, and salt.
- Add a sprinkle of paprika or a drizzle of olive oil to the hummus for a flavor boost.

Health Benefits

- Fiber: Carrots and cucumbers provide dietary fiber, aiding digestion and promoting satiety.
- Vitamins and Minerals: Hummus and vegetables are rich in vitamins and minerals, including vitamin A from carrots and vitamin K from cucumbers.

- Time of Preparation: 10 minutes
- Cooking Time: None
- Servings: 4

Ingredients

- 1 cup hummus (store-bought or homemade)
- 4 big carrots sliced into sticks after being peeled
- 2 cucumbers, sliced into sticks

Procedure

Prepare the carrots and cucumbers by peeling and cutting them into sticks.

3. Trail Mix with Nuts and Dried Fruits

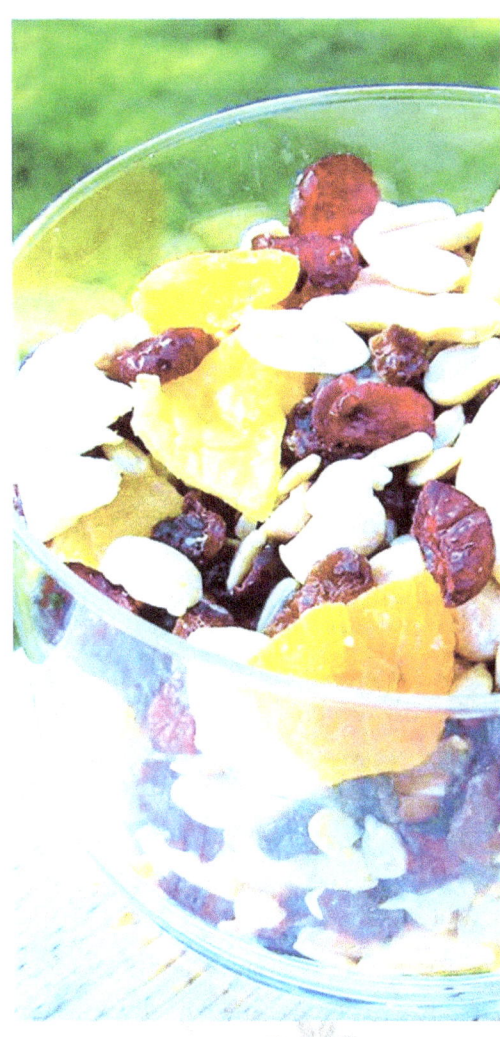

- Mix well to ensure an even distribution of nuts and dried fruits.
- Divide into small snack-sized portions or store in an airtight container.

Nutritional Values (per serving)

- Calories: 220
- Protein: 6g
- Carbohydrates: 20g
- Fiber: 4g
- Sugars: 12g
- Fat: 14g

Cooking Tips

- Use unsweetened dried fruits to reduce added sugars.
- Add dark chocolate chips or coconut flakes for extra flavor and texture.

Health Benefits

- Healthy Fats: Nuts and seeds provide healthy fats that support brain health.
- Antioxidants: Dried fruits like cranberries and apricots are rich in antioxidants, protecting cells from damage.

4. Baked Kale Chips

- Time of Preparation: 5 minutes
- Cooking Time: None
- Servings: 4

Ingredients

- 1/2 cup almonds
- 1/2 cup walnuts
- 1/2 cup dried cranberries
- 1/2 cup dried apricots, chopped
- 1/2 cup sunflower seeds

Procedure

- Combine all ingredients in a large bowl.

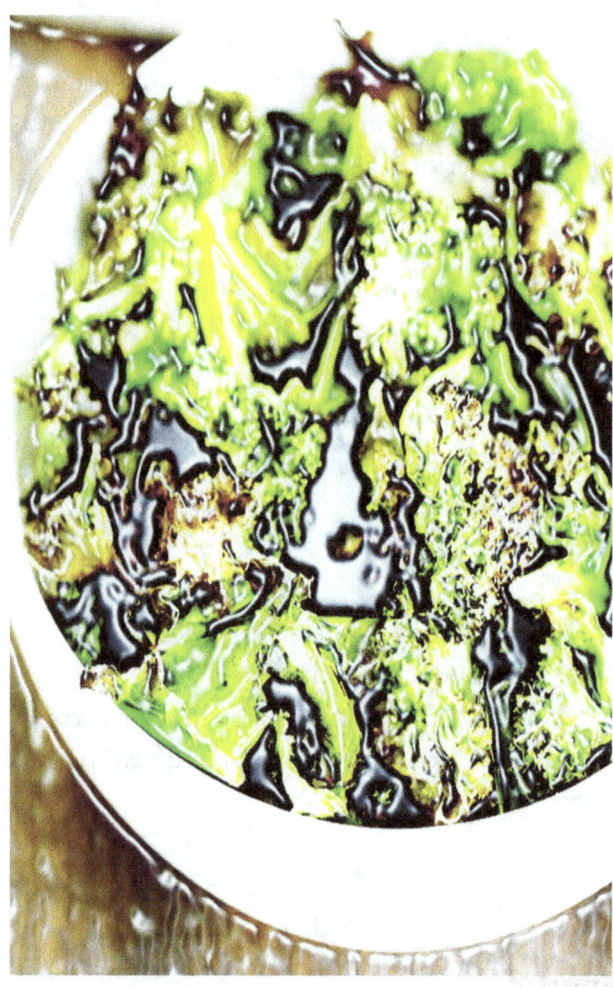

- Time of Preparation: 10 minutes
- Cooking Time: 20 minutes
- Servings: 4

Ingredients

- 1 bunch kale, washed and dried
- 2 tablespoons olive oil
- Salt to taste

Procedure

- Preheat the oven to 300°F (150°C).
- After heating, pick the kale leaves out and cut them into tiny pieces.
- Place the kale pieces in a large bowl, drizzle with olive oil, and sprinkle with salt.
- Massage the oil and salt into the kale to ensure even coating.
- Spread out the kale to form a single layer on a parchment paper-lined baking sheet.
- Bake for 15-20 minutes, turning once, until the edges are crispy and slightly browned.
- Let cool before serving.

Nutritional Values (per serving)

- Calories: 70
- Protein: 2g
- Carbohydrates: 5g
- Fiber: 2g
- Sugars: 1g
- Fat: 5g

Cooking Tips

- Ensure kale is completely dry before baking to achieve the best crispiness.
- Add spices like garlic powder, paprika, or nutritional yeast for added flavor.

Health Benefits

- Vitamins: Kale is an excellent source of vitamins A, C, and K, supporting immune and bone health.
- Antioxidants: Rich in antioxidants, kale helps protect against oxidative stress and inflammation.

5. Cottage Cheese with Pineapple Chunks

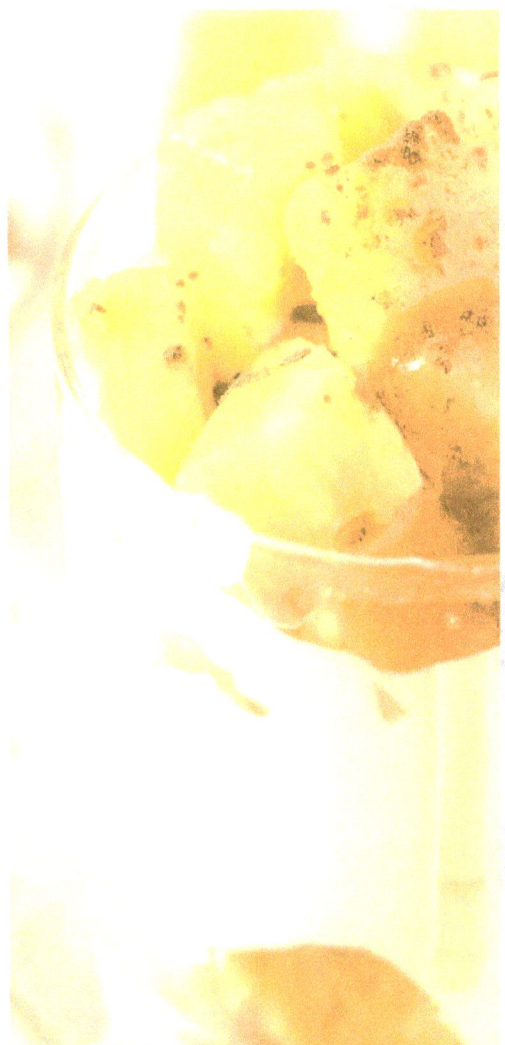

- Time of Preparation: 5 minutes
- Cooking Time: None
- Servings: 2

Ingredients

- 1 cup cottage cheese
- 1 cup fresh pineapple chunks

Procedure

- In a bowl, combine cottage cheese and pineapple chunks.
- Mix gently to combine.
- Proceed to serve it or store carefully in a refrigerator.

Nutritional Values (per serving)

- Calories: 150
- Protein: 14g
- Carbohydrates: 15g
- Fiber: 1g
- Sugars: 12g
- Fat: 4g

Cooking Tips

- Use fresh pineapple for the best flavor and texture, though canned pineapple (in juice, not syrup) can be used in a pinch.

Health Benefits

- **Protein:** Cottage cheese is high in protein, supporting muscle health and satiety.
- **Vitamins and Minerals:** Pineapple provides vitamin C and manganese, essential for immune function and bone health.

DR. JEFFREY M. WALTER

5 Dessert Recipes

Dessert Recipes: Sweet Treats for a Balanced Diet

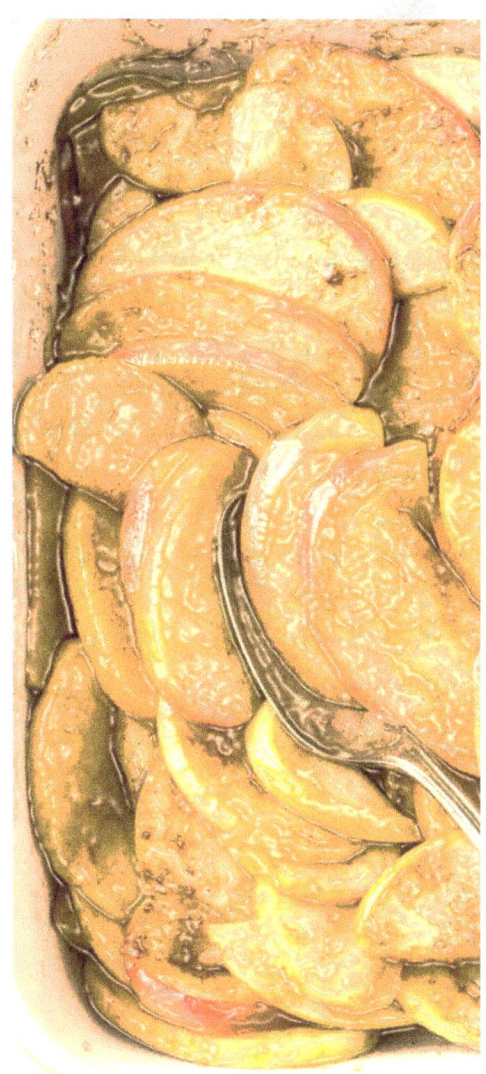

fresh fruits to create delicious desserts that seniors can enjoy without compromising their health.

Each recipe is designed to be easy to prepare and mindful of sugar and fat content, making them suitable for those managing Alzheimer's disease. From fruity delights to creamy indulgences, these desserts are the perfect way to end a meal on a high note.

Desserts can be a delightful part of a balanced diet, especially when made with wholesome ingredients. Our dessert recipes are crafted to offer a satisfying sweet treat while also providing nutritional benefits. These recipes use natural sweeteners, whole grains, and

DR. JEFFREY M. WALTER

1. Dark Chocolate and Nut Clusters

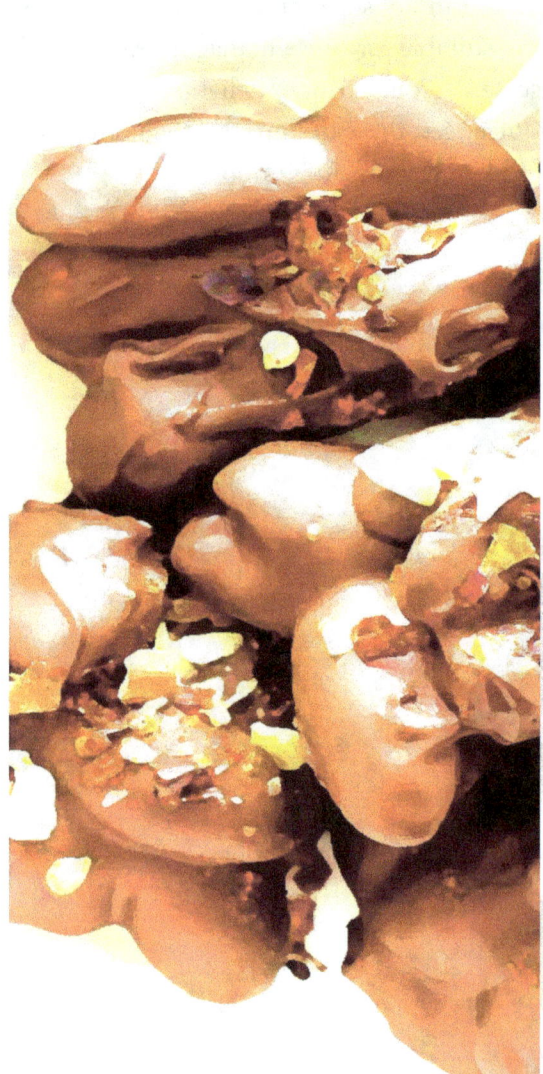

- Time of Preparation: 15 minutes
- Cooking Time: 10 minutes
- Servings: 12 clusters

Ingredients

- 8 oz dark chocolate (at least 70% cocoa), chopped
- 1 cup chopped mixed nuts (chopped cashews, walnuts, and almonds)
- Sea salt, for sprinkling (optional)

Procedure

- Line a baking sheet with parchment paper.
- The dark chocolate should be melted in a heatproof dish over a double boiler or in the microwave for 30-second bursts, stirring until smooth.
- Add the chopped nuts and stir until covered evenly.
- Drop tablespoon-sized clusters onto the baking sheet that has been ready.
- If desired, top with sea salt.
- The chocolate should set after approximately ten minutes in the refrigerator.
- Keep refrigerated in an airtight container.

Nutritional Values (per cluster)

- Calories: 120
- Protein: 2g
- Carbohydrates: 10g
- Fiber: 2g
- Sugars: 6g
- Fat: 8g

Cooking Tips

- Use a variety of nuts for different textures and flavors.
- Drizzle melted white chocolate over the clusters for a decorative touch.

Health Benefits

- Antioxidants: Dark chocolate is rich in antioxidants, which help protect cells from damage.
- Healthy Fats: Nuts provide healthy fats that support heart health and cognitive function.

2. Baked Apples with Cinnamon

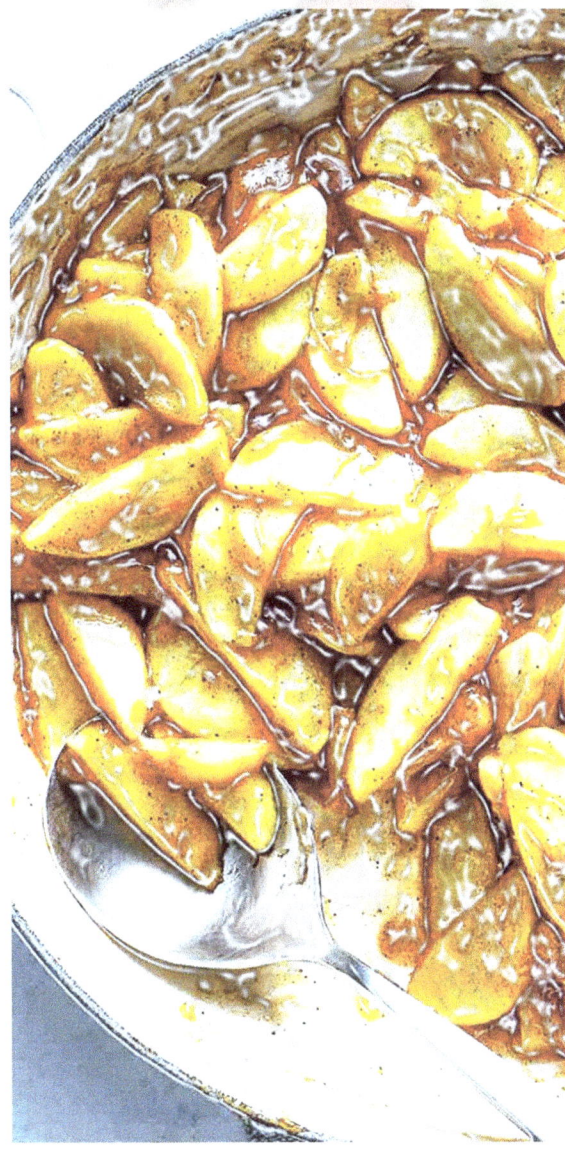

- Time of Preparation: 10 minutes
- Cooking Time: 30 minutes
- Servings: 4

Ingredients

- 4 large apples (such as Granny Smith or Honeycrisp), cored
- 1/4 cup raisins or dried cranberries
- 2 tablespoons chopped nuts (pecans or walnuts)
- 2 tablespoons honey or maple syrup
- 1 teaspoon ground cinnamon
- 1/4 cup water

Procedure

- Preheat the oven to 375°F (190°C).
- In a small bowl, mix together raisins or dried cranberries, chopped nuts, honey or maple syrup, and ground cinnamon.
- Stuff each cored apple with the mixture and place in a baking dish.
- Fill the baking dish's bottom with water.
- Bake the apples for 25 to 30 minutes, or until they are soft.
- Serve hot

Nutritional Values (per serving)

- Calories: 180
- Protein: 2g
- Carbohydrates: 40g
- Fiber: 6g
- Sugars: 30g
- Fat: 4g

Cooking Tips

- Pick apples that bake up well in terms of form.
- Change the quantity of honey or maple syrup to adjust the sweetness.
- Benefits to Health: Dietary fiber, which helps digestive health, is found in apples.
- Vitamins and Minerals: Cinnamon adds flavor and may have anti-inflammatory properties.

3. Greek Yogurt Parfait with Honey and Nut

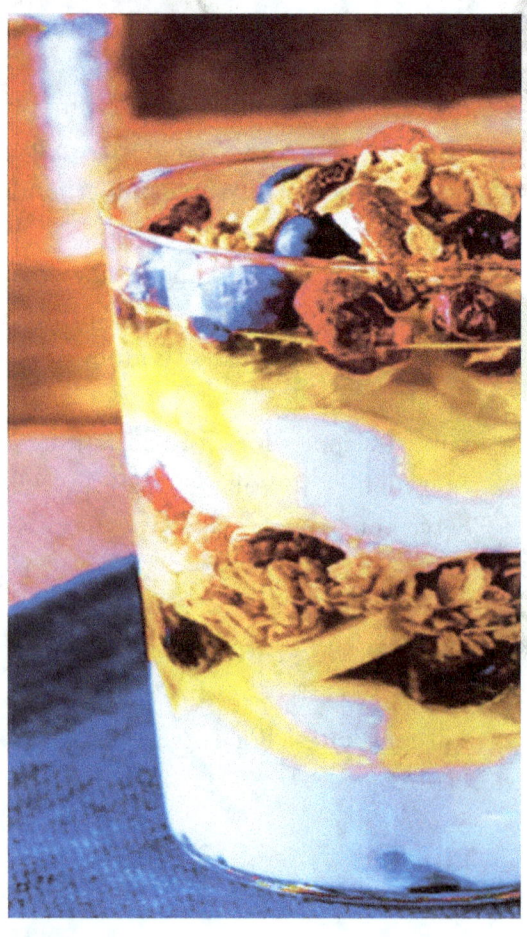

- Time of Preparation: 5 minutes
- Cooking Time: None
- Servings: 2

Ingredients

- 1 cup Greek yogurt
- 2 tablespoons honey
- 1/4 cup chopped nuts (almonds, walnuts, pecans)
- Fresh berries (optional)

Procedure

- In two serving glasses or bowls, layer Greek yogurt, honey, and chopped nuts.
- Repeat layers until ingredients are used up.
- Top with fresh berries if desired.
- Serve immediately.

Nutritional Values (per serving)

- Calories: 250
- Protein: 20g
- Carbohydrates: 20g
- Fiber: 2g
- Sugars: 18g
- Fat: 12g

Cooking Tips

- Use plain Greek yogurt for a tangy contrast to the sweetness of honey and berries.
- Add granola or toasted oats for additional texture.

Health Benefits

- Protein: Greek yogurt is high in protein, supporting muscle health and satiety.
- Antioxidants: Nuts and berries provide antioxidants that help protect against oxidative stress.

4. Fresh Berry Salad with Mint

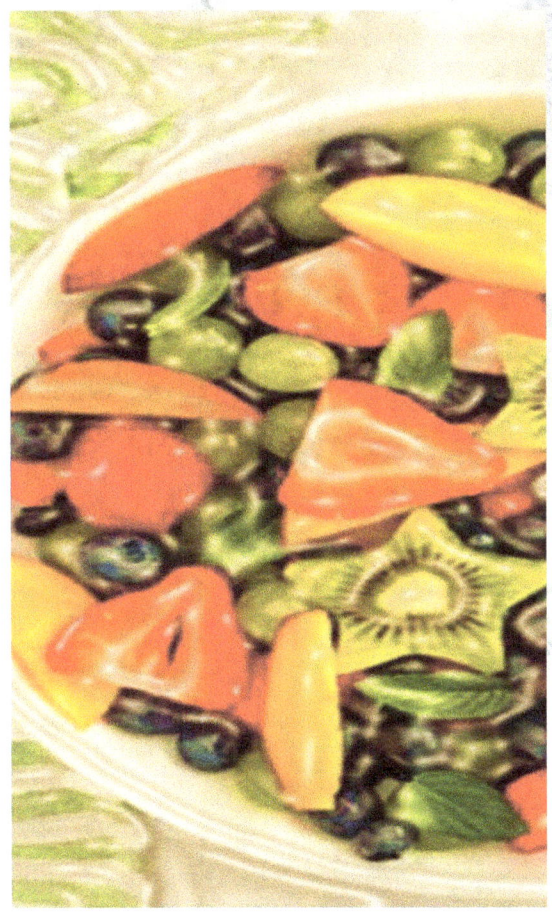

- Time of preparation: 10 minutes
- Cooking Time: None
- Servings: 4

Ingredients

- Two cups of assorted fresh berries.
- 1 tablespoon fresh mint leaves, chopped
- 1 tablespoon honey or maple syrup
- 1 teaspoon lemon juice
- Optional: Greek yogurt or whipped cream for serving

Procedure

- In a large bowl, gently toss together fresh berries, chopped mint leaves, honey or maple syrup, and lemon juice.
- Wait for a few minutes.
- Serve in individual bowls or glasses.
- Optional: Serve with a dollop of Greek yogurt or whipped cream on top.

Nutritional Values (per serving)

- Calories: 60
- Protein: 1g
- Carbohydrates: 15g
- Fiber: 3g

- Sugars: 11g
- Fat: 0g

Cooking Tips

- Use a variety of berries for different colors and flavors.
- Adjust sweetness with more or less honey or maple syrup.

Health Benefits

- Vitamins: Berries contain vitamin C, which supports immune function and skin health.
- Low-Calorie: This dessert option is low in calories but high in flavor and nutrients.

5. Banana Oat Cookies

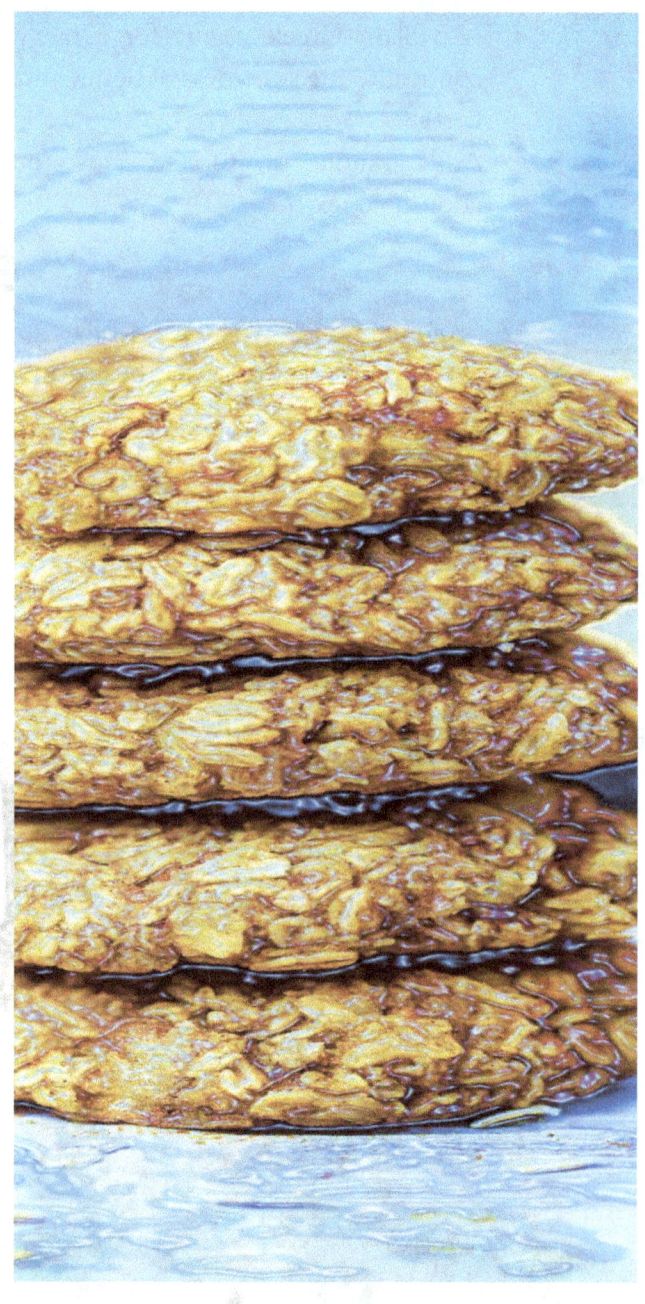

- Time of Preparation: 10 minutes
- Cooking Time: 15 minutes
- Servings: 12 cookies

Ingredients

- 2 ripe bananas, mashed
- 1 cup rolled oats
- 1/4 cup chopped nuts (walnuts or almonds)
- 1/4 cup dried cranberries or raisins
- 1 teaspoon ground cinnamon
- 1/4 teaspoon vanilla extract

Procedure

- Preheat the oven to 350°F (175°C). Line a baking sheet with parchment paper.
- In a mixing bowl, combine mashed bananas, rolled oats, chopped nuts, dried cranberries or raisins, cinnamon, and vanilla extract. Mix well.
- Drop spoonfuls of the mixture onto the prepared baking sheet, shaping into cookies with the back of the spoon.
- Bake, or until golden brown, about 15 minutes.
- Before serving, take out of the oven and let it cool on a wire rack.

Nutritional Values (per cookie)

- Calories: 90
- Protein: 2g
- Carbohydrates: 15g
- Fiber: 2g
- Sugars: 7g
- Fat: 3g

Cooking Tips

- Add chocolate chips or coconut flakes for added sweetness and texture.

Health Benefits

- Whole Grains: Rolled oats provide fiber that supports digestive health.
- Potassium: Bananas are a good source of potassium, which helps maintain healthy blood pressure.
- Natural Sweeteners: Bananas and dried fruit add sweetness without refined sugars.

6 Beverage Recipes

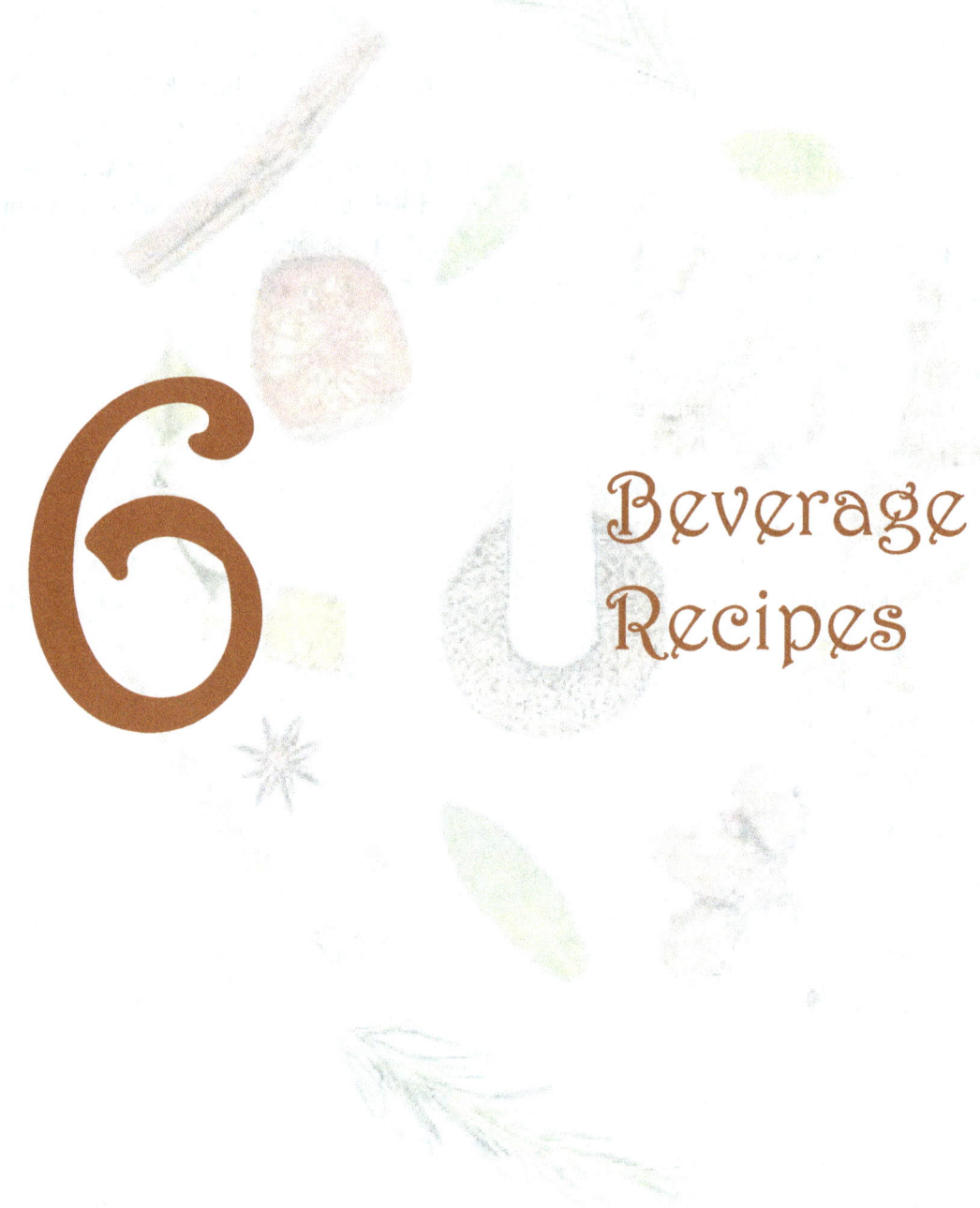

DR. JEFFREY M. WALTER

Beverages: Refreshing and Nourishing Drinks

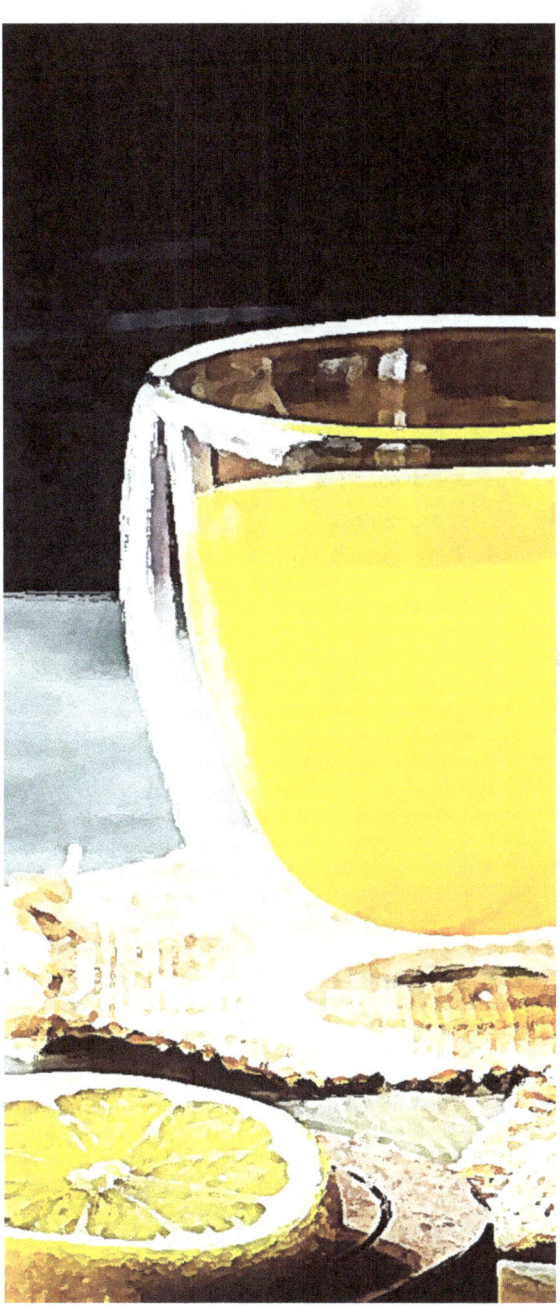

Beverages play a vital role in hydration and can complement a nutritious diet for seniors managing Alzheimer's disease. Our beverage selections focus on providing refreshing options that are easy to prepare and packed with health benefits.

From hydrating fruit-infused waters to soothing herbal teas, our recipes are designed to cater to different tastes and preferences while promoting overall well-being. Whether enjoyed with meals or as a standalone refreshment, these beverages ensure seniors stay hydrated and nourished throughout the day.

DR. JEFFREY M. WALTER

1. Green Tea with Lemon

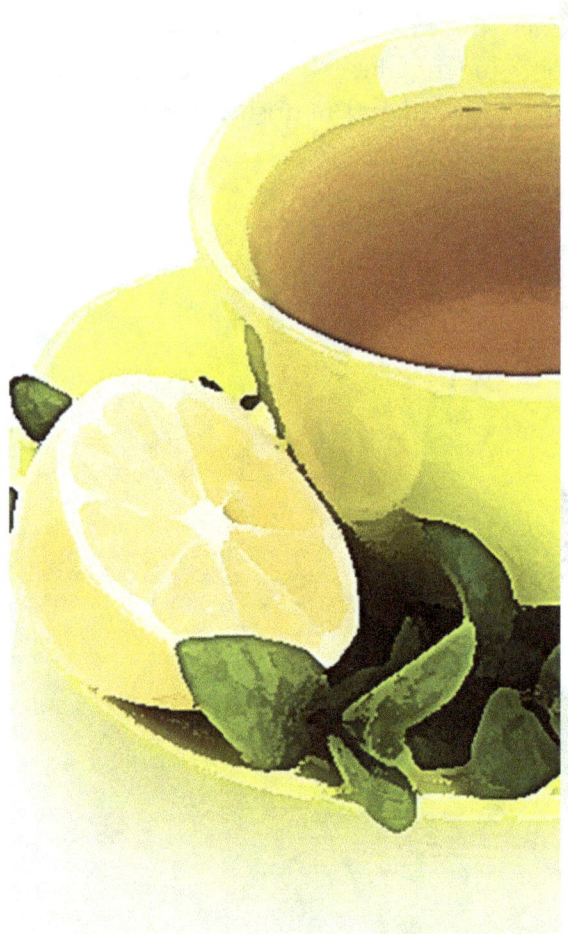

- Cooking Time: 5 minutes
- Servings: 2

Ingredients

- 2 cups water
- 2 green tea bags
- 1 lemon, sliced
- Honey or stevia (optional, for sweetness)

Procedure

- Transfer the water in a small saucepan to a boil.
- Take off the heat and put the green tea bags in.
- Based on the desired strength, steep for three to five minutes.
- Remove tea bags and pour tea into serving cups.
- Add lemon slices and sweeten with honey or stevia if desired.
- Stir well and serve hot or chilled over ice.

Nutritional Values (per serving)

- Calories: 0
- Protein: 0g
- Carbohydrates: 0g
- Fiber: 0g
- Sugars: 0g
- Fat: 0g

Cooking Tips

- Do not over steep green tea to avoid bitterness.
- Use fresh lemon for the best flavor and vitamin C content.

Health Benefits

- Time of Preparation: 5 minutes

- Antioxidants: Green tea is rich in antioxidants, which help protect cells from damage.
- Caffeine: Provides a gentle boost of caffeine for alertness without the jitters.

2. Berry Infused Water

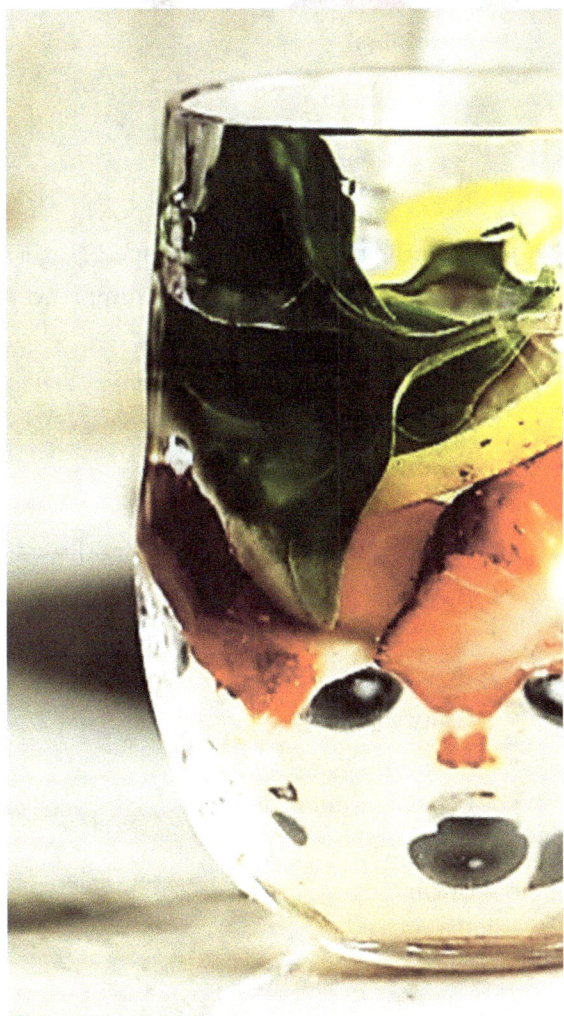

- Time of Preparation: 5 minutes
- Cooking Time: None
- Servings: 4

Ingredients

- One cup of freshly mixed berries
- 1 lemon, thinly sliced
- 4 cups water
- Ice cubes

Procedure

- Add both lemon slices and mixed berries.
- Pour water over the berries and lemon.
- Refrigerate for at least 1 hour to allow flavors to infuse.
- Serve chilled over ice.

Nutritional Values (per serving)

- Calories: 10
- Protein: 0g
- Carbohydrates: 3g
- Fiber: 1g
- Sugars: 1g
- Fat: 0g

Cooking Tips

- Crush berries slightly before adding to release more flavor.

Health Benefits

- Hydration: Infused water encourages increased water intake, essential for overall health.
- Vitamins and Antioxidants: Berries and lemon provide vitamins and antioxidants that support immune function.

3. Ginger and Turmeric Tea

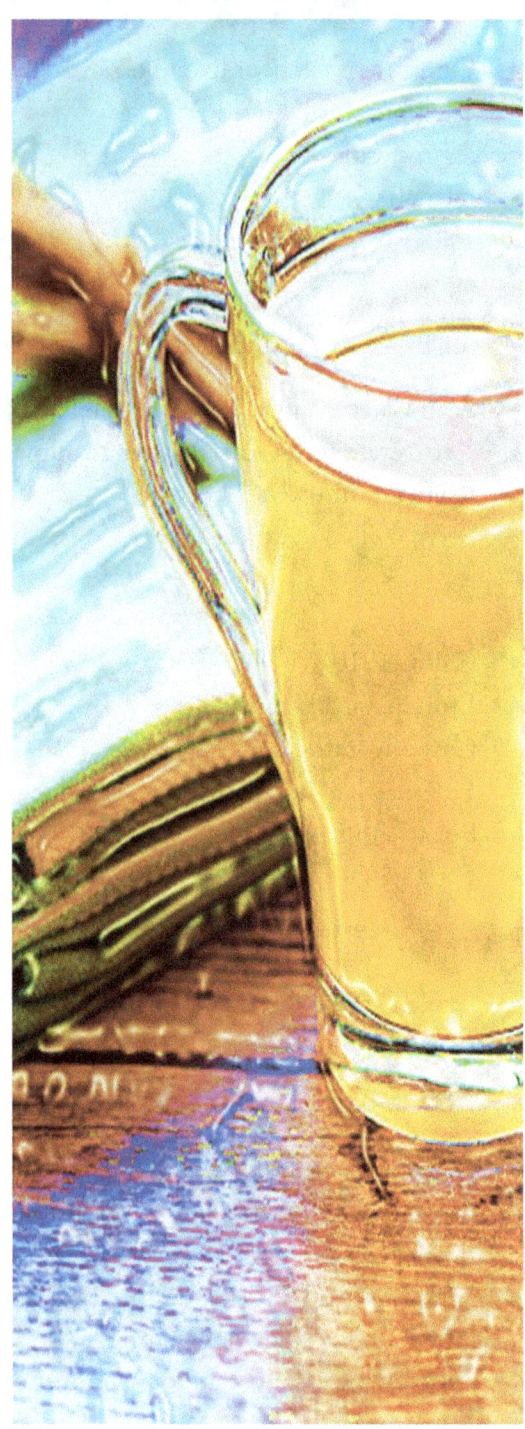

- Time of Preparation: 10 minutes
- Cooking Time: 10 minutes
- Servings: 2

Ingredients

- 2 cups water
- 1-inch piece ginger, peeled and thinly sliced
- 1 teaspoon ground turmeric or 1-inch piece fresh turmeric, thinly sliced
- 1 tablespoon honey (optional, for sweetness)
- Lemon wedges (optional, for garnish)

Procedure

- Boil some water in a small pot.
- Add the turmeric and chopped ginger.
- For five to ten minutes, simmer over low heat.
- Take off the heat and steep for five more minutes.
- Strain tea into serving cups.
- Stir in honey if desired.
- Garnish with lemon wedges and serve hot.

Nutritional Values (per serving)

- Calories: 10
- Protein: 0g
- Carbohydrates: 3g
- Fiber: 0g
- Sugars: 3g
- Fat: 0g

Cooking Tips

- Adjust ginger and turmeric to taste, as they can vary in potency.
- Use fresh turmeric for a more vibrant color and flavor.

Health Benefits

- Anti-inflammatory: Ginger and turmeric have anti-inflammatory properties that may help reduce inflammation in the body.
- Digestive Aid: Ginger can aid digestion and alleviate nausea.
- Antioxidants: Turmeric contains curcumin, a powerful antioxidant that supports overall health.

4. Fresh Vegetable Juice Blend

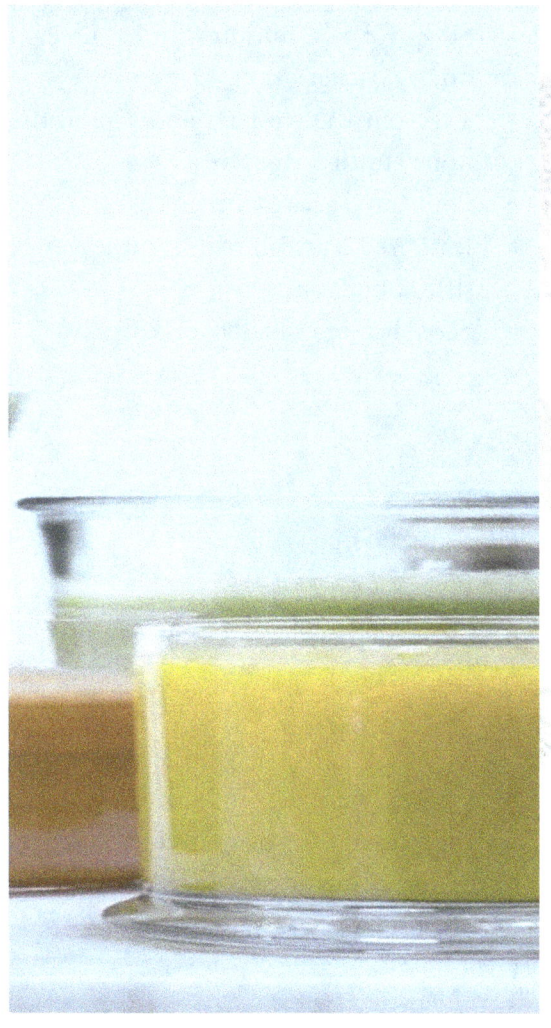

- Time of Preparation: 10 minutes
- Cooking Time: None
- Servings: 2

Ingredients

- 2 large carrots, washed and trimmed
- 2 stalks celery, washed
- 1 cucumber, washed
- 1 small beet, washed and peeled
- 1 lemon, peeled

Procedure

- Cut vegetables and lemon into sizes that will fit into your juicer chute.
- Juice the carrots, celery, cucumber, beet, and lemon according to your juicer's instructions.
- Stir well to combine.
- Serve chilled

Nutritional Values (per serving)

- Calories: 80
- Protein: 2g
- Carbohydrates: 18g
- Fiber: 4g
- Sugars: 10g
- Fat: 0g

Cooking Tips

- Adjust the vegetable quantities to suit your taste preferences.
- Add a dash of cayenne pepper or ginger for an extra kick.

Health Benefits

- Vitamins and Minerals: Provides a concentrated source of vitamins A, C, and K from the vegetables.
- Hydration: Juices help hydrate the body and replenish electrolytes.
- Antioxidants: Carotenoids from carrots and betalains from beets offer antioxidant benefits.

5. Herbal Tea with Honey

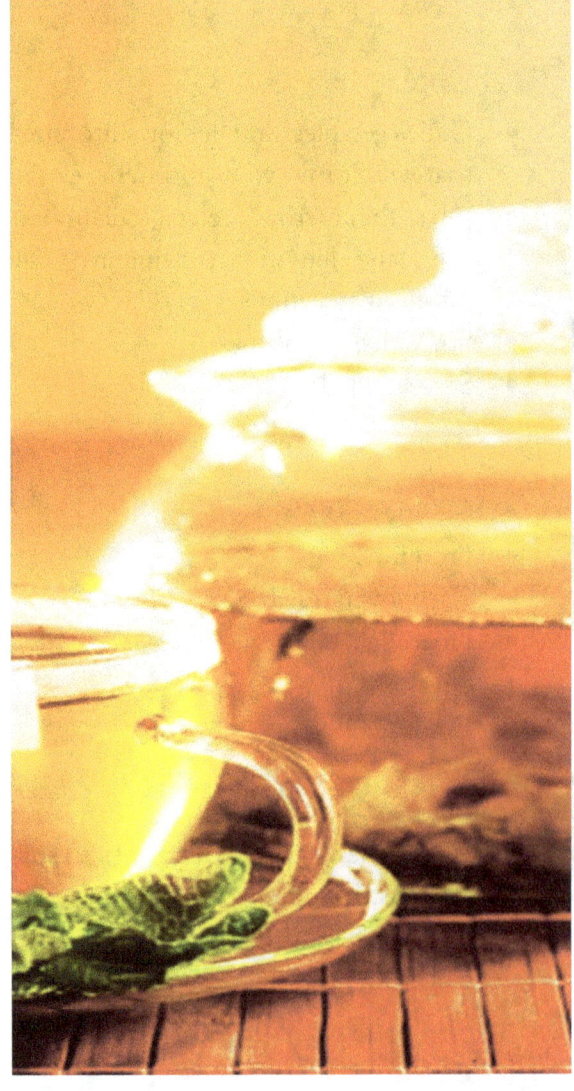

- Time of Preparation: 5 minutes
- Cooking Time: 5 minutes
- Servings: 2

Ingredients

- 2 cups water
- 2 herbal tea bags (such as chamomile, peppermint, or rooibos)
- 1 tablespoon honey
- Garnish with optional lemon slices or mint leaves.

Procedure

- Transfer the water in a small saucepan to a boil.
- Take off the heat and put the herbal tea bags in.
- Steep for five minutes, or as directed on the packet.
- Take out the tea bags and mix in the honey until it dissolves.
- Pour into serving cups.
- If desired, garnish with mint leaves or slices of lemon.
- Serve hot or chilled over ice.

Nutritional Values (per serving)

- Calories: 20
- Protein: 0g
- Carbohydrates: 5g
- Fiber: 0g
- Sugars: 5g
- Fat: 0g

Cooking Tips

- Choose herbal teas known for their calming or digestive properties.
- Adjust sweetness by adding more or less honey.

Health Benefits

- Relaxation: Herbal teas like chamomile promote relaxation and may help with sleep.
- Digestive Aid: Peppermint tea can aid digestion and alleviate bloating.
- Antioxidants: Rooibos tea is rich in antioxidants that support immune health.

DR. JEFFREY M. WALTER

7 Meal Plan

DR. JEFFREY M. WALTER

Meal Plan

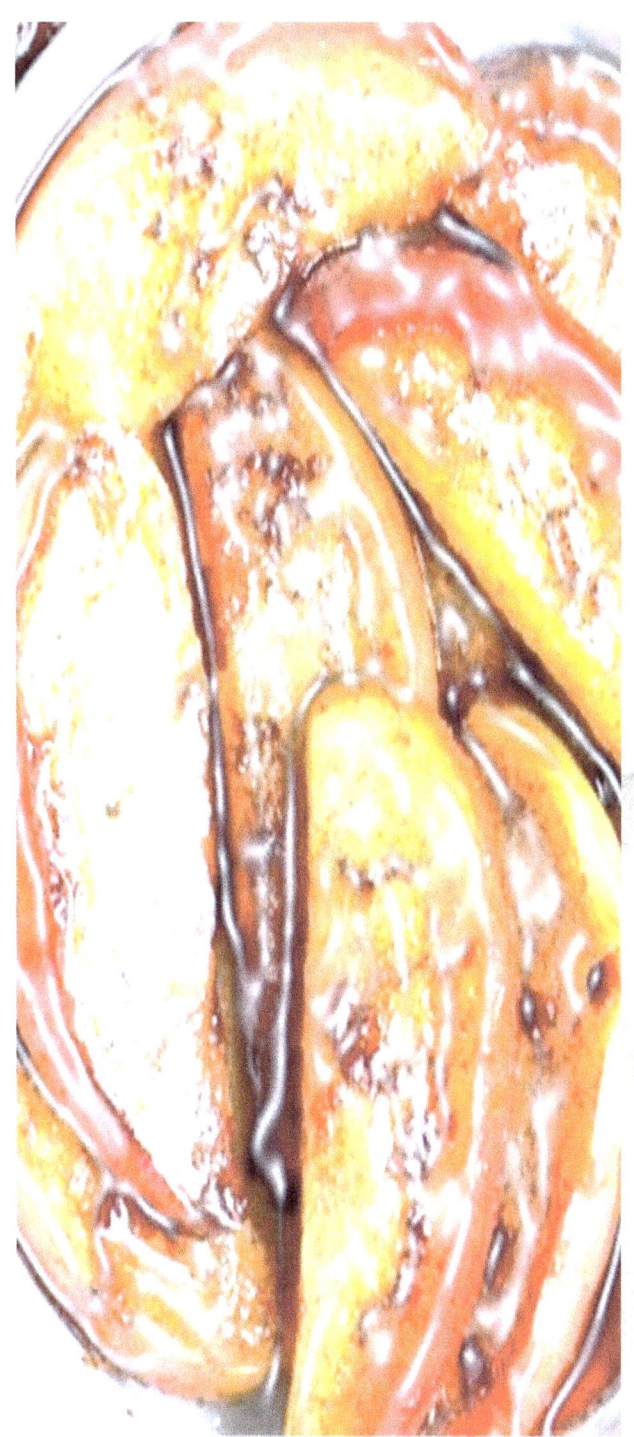

Creating a well-structured meal plan is essential for ensuring that seniors with Alzheimer's disease receive balanced and nutritious meals consistently. This meal plan provides a comprehensive guide to crafting daily and weekly meal plans that incorporate a variety of recipes from different categories, including breakfast, lunch, dinner, snacks, and beverages.

Each meal plan is designed to offer a harmonious blend of essential nutrients, focusing on foods that support cognitive health and overall well-being.

With a thoughtful combination of fruits, vegetables, lean proteins, whole grains, and healthy fats, these meal plans aim to maintain energy levels, support brain function, and promote physical health.

By following the meal plans provided, caregivers can simplify the process of meal preparation and ensure that their loved ones enjoy a diverse and delicious diet.

Each plan includes easy-to-follow recipes, clear preparation and cooking times, and detailed nutritional information, making it easier to manage dietary needs and preferences.

Whether you are preparing meals for a day or planning for the week ahead, this book equips you with the tools to create balanced and satisfying menus.

From hearty breakfasts to nourishing dinners, and refreshing beverages to tasty snacks, every meal is an opportunity to provide care and support through wholesome food.

By integrating these meal plans into daily routines, caregivers can help enhance the quality of life for seniors with Alzheimer's, ensuring they receive the nutrition they need to thrive.

DR. JEFFREY M. WALTER

14-Days Meal Plan

Here is a 14 days meal plan for seniors with Alzheimer's disease,

Week 1
Day 1
Breakfast: Blueberry Oatmeal with Walnuts
Lunch: Quinoa Salad with Kale and Cranberries
Dinner: Baked Salmon with Asparagus
Snack: Apple Slices with Almond Butter
Dessert: Dark Chocolate and Nut Clusters
Beverage: Green Tea with Lemon
Day 2
Breakfast: Spinach and Mushroom Frittata
Lunch: Lentil Soup with Carrots and Celery
Dinner: Chicken and Vegetable Stir-Fry
Snack: Hummus with Carrot and Cucumber Sticks
Dessert: Baked Apples with Cinnamon
Beverage: Berry Infused Water
Day 3
Breakfast: Avocado and Berry Smoothie
Lunch: Grilled Chicken and Avocado Wrap
Dinner: Stuffed Bell Peppers with Brown Rice
Snack: Trail Mix with Nuts and Dried Fruits
Dessert: Greek Yogurt Parfait with Honey and Nuts
Beverage: Ginger and Turmeric Tea
Day 4
Breakfast: Greek Yogurt with Honey and Almonds
Lunch: Roasted Beet and Goat Cheese Salad
Dinner: Herb-Crusted Cod with Quinoa
Snack: Baked Kale Chips
Dessert: Fresh Berry Salad with Mint
Beverage: Fresh Vegetable Juice Blend
Day 5
Breakfast: Chia Seed Pudding with Fresh Berries
Lunch: Tomato Basil Soup with Whole Grain Bread
Dinner: Sweet Potato and Black Bean Enchiladas
Snack: Cottage Cheese with Pineapple Chunks
Dessert: Banana Oat Cookies
Beverage: Herbal Tea with Honey
Day 6
Breakfast: Blueberry Oatmeal with Walnuts
Lunch: Quinoa Salad with Kale and Cranberries
Dinner: Baked Salmon with Asparagus
Snack: Apple Slices with Almond Butter
Dessert: Dark Chocolate and Nut Clusters
Beverage: Green Tea with Lemon
Day 7
Breakfast: Spinach and Mushroom Frittata
Lunch: Lentil Soup with Carrots and Celery
Dinner: Chicken and Vegetable Stir-Fry
Snack: Hummus with Carrot and Cucumber Sticks
Dessert: Baked Apples with Cinnamon
Beverage: Berry Infused Water
Week 2
Day 8
Breakfast: Avocado and Berry Smoothie
Lunch: Grilled Chicken and Avocado Wrap
Dinner: Stuffed Bell Peppers with Brown Rice
Snack: Trail Mix with Nuts and Dried Fruits
Dessert: Greek Yogurt Parfait with Honey and Nuts
Beverage: Ginger and Turmeric Tea
Day 9
Breakfast: Greek Yogurt with Honey and Almonds
Lunch: Roasted Beet and Goat Cheese Salad
Dinner: Herb-Crusted Cod with Quinoa
Snack: Baked Kale Chips
Dessert: Fresh Berry Salad with Mint
Beverage: Fresh Vegetable Juice Blend
Day 10
Breakfast: Chia Seed Pudding with Fresh Berries
Lunch: Tomato Basil Soup with Whole Grain Bread
Dinner: Sweet Potato and Black Bean Enchiladas

Snack: Cottage Cheese with Pineapple Chunks
Dessert: Banana Oat Cookies
Beverage: Herbal Tea with Honey
Day 11
Breakfast: Blueberry Oatmeal with Walnuts
Lunch: Quinoa Salad with Kale and Cranberries
Dinner: Baked Salmon with Asparagus
Snack: Apple Slices with Almond Butter
Dessert: Dark Chocolate and Nut Clusters
Beverage: Green Tea with Lemon
Day 12
Breakfast: Spinach and Mushroom Frittata
Lunch: Lentil Soup with Carrots and Celery
Dinner: Chicken and Vegetable Stir-Fry
Snack: Hummus with Carrot and Cucumber Sticks
Dessert: Baked Apples with Cinnamon
Beverage: Berry Infused Water
Day 13
Breakfast: Avocado and Berry Smoothie
Lunch: Grilled Chicken and Avocado Wrap
Dinner: Stuffed Bell Peppers with Brown Rice
Snack: Trail Mix with Nuts and Dried Fruits
Dessert: Greek Yogurt Parfait with Honey and Nuts
Beverage: Ginger and Turmeric Tea
Day 14
Breakfast: Greek Yogurt with Honey and Almonds
Lunch: Roasted Beet and Goat Cheese Salad
Dinner: Herb-Crusted Cod with Quinoa
Snack: Baked Kale Chips
Dessert: Fresh Berry Salad with Mint
Beverage: Fresh Vegetable Juice Blend

This 14-day meal plan provides a balanced variety of nutrient-rich recipes designed to support cognitive health and overall well-being for seniors managing Alzheimer's disease. By following this plan, caregivers can ensure their loved ones receive delicious, nutritious meals every day.

DR. JEFFREY M. WALTER

Advice for Seniors and Families

Embracing Each Day with Positivity
Life is a journey filled with countless moments of joy, learning, and growth. As we navigate the challenges and triumphs that come with aging and caring for loved ones, it's essential to embrace each day with a positive outlook. Every sunrise offers a new opportunity to cherish the simple pleasures, celebrate the small victories, and create beautiful memories with those we love.

- The Power of Resilience

Seniors, with their wealth of experiences and wisdom, embody resilience. They have weathered many storms and emerged stronger, teaching us the invaluable lesson that it's not about how many times we fall, but how many times we rise. Families, too, show remarkable resilience as they support their loved ones through life's challenges. Together, we can find strength in unity and hope in perseverance.

- Celebrating the Moments That Matter

Life's most precious moments are often the simplest ones: a shared meal, a heartfelt conversation, a walk in the park. These moments remind us of the importance of being present and appreciating the here and now.

For seniors and their families, it's about making the most of the time spent together, cherishing every laugh, every hug, and every word of wisdom shared.

- The Gift of Love and Care

Caring for a loved one, especially those with Alzheimer's, is an act of profound love and compassion. It is a testament to the bonds that hold families together. As caregivers, your dedication and unwavering support make a world of difference.

Remember that your efforts, no matter how small they may seem, are invaluable. The love and care you provide are the greatest gifts of all.

- Finding Joy in Everyday Activities

Joy can be found in the everyday activities that bring us together. Whether it's cooking a meal from this cookbook, reminiscing over old photographs, or simply enjoying a cup of tea, these moments are opportunities to connect and find happiness. Embrace these activities with a light heart and an open mind, allowing them to bring warmth and joy into your lives.

- Hope for the Future

While Alzheimer's presents its challenges, it also brings families closer and highlights the importance of hope and optimism. Advances in research and a growing understanding of the disease offer hope for better treatments and care. As we look to the future, let's remain hopeful and supportive of one another, knowing that each day brings new possibilities and opportunities for connection and love.

- **Together, We Thrive**

The journey of aging and caregiving is not one that must be traveled alone. Together, seniors and their families can find strength, comfort, and joy in each other's company. By supporting one another, sharing in the ups and downs, and celebrating the moments that truly matter, we can create a tapestry of love and resilience that enriches our lives and the lives of those around us.

Wrapping up

An appropriately balanced diet is essential for maintaining general health, cognitive function, and older citizens' quality of life while managing Alzheimer's disease. We've looked at a range of recipes in this cookbook that are meant to provide tasty, nutrient-dense meals and snacks that also happen to be good for brain health.

Every cuisine, from breakfast to supper, as well as decadent desserts and reviving drinks, has been developed using components that are recognized to enhance general well-being and cognitive performance.

Motivation to Maintain a Healthy Diet

Keeping up a healthy diet is a journey that calls for dedication and perseverance. A healthy diet has advantages for elders with Alzheimer's disease that go beyond physical health to improve mental and emotional well-being.

As family members and caregivers, you may have a big influence on the everyday lives of the people you look for by supporting them in developing healthy eating habits.

You can make sure that every meal is a step toward enhancing brain health and general vigor by adding these recipes to regular meal plans and customizing them to suit individual tastes and dietary requirements.

Last words of advice for caregivers

Diverse and adaptable: To guarantee a nutritionally balanced diet, embrace variation in your meal planning. Be adaptable and modify recipes to suit dietary requirements and personal tastes.

Encourage proper hydration throughout the day by sipping on water and nutrient-rich drinks like fresh juices and herbal teas.

Patience and Understanding: Recognize that eating habits may change as Alzheimer's progresses, and approach meals with patience and understanding. Establish a relaxing and cozy setting to encourage pleasurable eating experiences.

Consultation with healthcare specialists: For individualized nutritional advice and assistance catered to specific requirements, always contact healthcare specialists, such as registered dietitians.

Mealtimes are a wonderful time to interact and have fun. Make the most of them. Eat meals together, converse with one another, and enjoy the benefits of food as a source of happiness and sustenance.

Remember that every meal you cook with love and purpose for your loved ones with Alzheimer's disease improves their general health as you continue on this road of providing care and support.

DR. JEFFREY M. WALTER

Working together, we can harness the power of wholesome and delectable cuisine to enable seniors to flourish.

www.ingramcontent.com/pod-product-compliance
Lightning Source LLC
Chambersburg PA
CBHW082239220526
45479CB00005B/1281